HUMBLE PIE

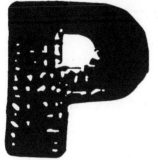
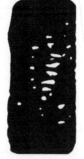
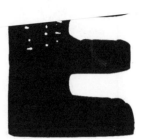

**WRITTEN
BY
PAT
LaMARCHE**

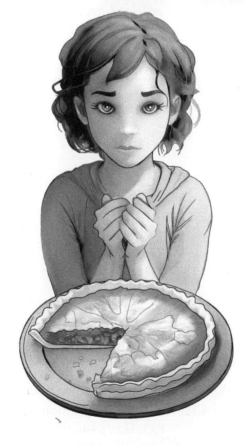

**ILLUSTRATED
BY
JEREMY
RUBY**

FEATURING SPECIALTY RECIPES BY CHEF ARCHIE

Charles Bruce Foundation
Carlisle, Pennsylvania

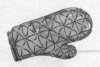

The recipes listed in this book are creations belonging to the individuals who contributed them. Any similarity to otherwise published recipes is a matter of coincidence.

This book commemorates the needless
suffering experienced by hungry people.

Table of Contents

Preface

First things first – this is not a definitive book on cooking, eating or nutrition. Nor is it a compendium for, or commentary on, gastronomical delights. Oh sure, some of the recipes in this book, when followed properly, will yield a tasty treat.

That said, fortunately for you, I have a friend who is a European chef. Whenever you see a QR code alongside a recipe, it will take you to a video on his YouTube channel. If you like to cook and eat, you will not be disappointed. His recipes and a number of others from some amateur chefs will make this a valuable addition to your kitchen. Meanwhile, what I'm really after is your heart.

Like most of my books, I'm hoping to catch your attention. The recipes are a hook. You'll find them scattered among a collection of personal accounts, peppered with heart-wrenching tales of folks who encounter adversity and how they survive – or thrive – or not.

In *Humble Pie* you will find my private observations, individual and family recollections. As a journalist, I've included research where it seems germane. You'll read cautionary narratives about poverty and neglect. I think you'll marvel, as I did, at the agility some folks exhibit when dealing with daily strife. Because what I write can be difficult to read, I've interspersed these truthful tales with recipes from the front line. You'll be dumbfounded, no doubt, at the ingenuity displayed by those who struggled to feed themselves and their families.

Many of the recipes are delicious. Others are haphazard, spartan or cobbled together from barely palatable ingredients. Necessity or privation (or both) cause these culinary creations to be fondly recalled and therefore still "taste good" – even today – to those who nostalgically prepare them. Nearly all the meals detailed here were warmly received at the time, regardless of flavor, because, as Ben Franklin noted, "Hunger is the best sauce."

In addition to the stories and recipes, I'll *pepper* the book (see what I did there?) with more general facts. In the back you will find a bibliography of my resources. Feel free to poke around the websites mentioned there. You'll find a wealth of knowledge and countless information-laden rabbit holes through which to fall.

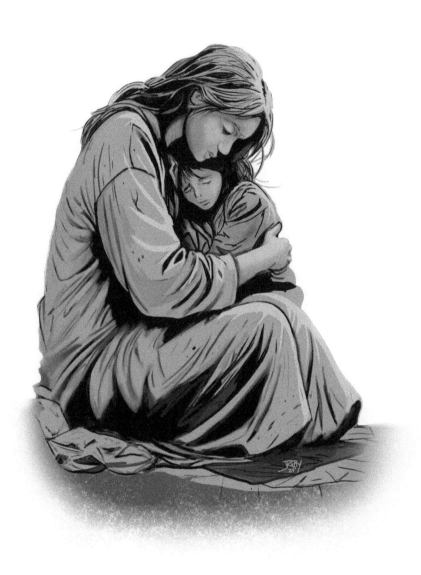

Food: It's Personal

Introduction

I find it interesting that there's enough wealth in the world for some people to have golden toilet seats, but not enough for vast multitudes to have spinach. The argument might be made that toilet seats and spinach both imply comfort or status. Depending on one's reality, both are difficult to acquire. In July of 2021, *Slate Magazine* fixed the price of an 18-carat-gold-plated toilet at $22,000. That one elaborate commode would've paid for 62,858 kilos of spinach in Ghana – enough for more than half a million people to have 250 grams each (roughly half a pound).

While one may survive without a commode of precious metals, food remains essential. And despite the obscene frivolity of golden toilets, this extravagance pales when compared to the largesse wasted by the industrial world's investment in the military industrial complex. No matter the source of the wasted resource, opulence or armaments, it's all irrelevant. The point remains that, for some people in the world, basic nutrition is a scarce commodity – a luxury, even.

While writing this book, I interviewed a Syrian refugee who had emigrated to Gander, Newfoundland. He, his wife and children journeyed to this small town as part of a Canadian program to remedy falling population rates by bringing refugees of war to safety. Agonizingly, the refugee family left their extended family behind – in a country where the only fecund food scavenging is done in hospital dumpsters.

According to the website, *The World Counts*, nine million people die each year – and have died each year since the century began – of starvation. The same site proclaims that one in nine persons go to bed each night hungry. Of course, *The World Counts* is a global website based in Copenhagen, Denmark. Their figures include statistics from many exceptionally hungry places in the world – think sub-Saharan Africa and extremely desolate parts of Asia. What bears noting, though, is that the percentage of hungry people worldwide is the same as the percentage of hungry people in the United States. Wouldn't you have thought the odds of being well fed would be better in the wealthiest nation on the planet?

Feeding America, an organization that focuses primarily on the U.S., cites the same statistics. Forty million hungry people in the U.S. – out of roughly 334 million. If you're doing the math at home, that's closer to one in eight – a little worse than one in nine.

So, the U.S. is a perfect example of the world in general. The U.S. is a region on the globe with concentrated wealth surrounded by – frankly – a third world. First world, third world: we got it all – right here. The myth that starvation and malnutrition are signaled only by babies with swollen bellies and flies on their eyes is proven false by any number of American barometers. The U.S. infant mortality rate is one.

The *CIA (U.S. Central Intelligence Agency) World Fact Book* places the infant mortality rates here in the United States just after Serbia, Bosnia Herzegovina, and United Arab Emirates. We are outpacing less-competitive locations such as New Caledonia, Latvia and Slovakia, respectively. In case you were wondering … the U.S. is twelve places behind Cuba. Seventeen behind Lithuania. Twenty-six behind Belarus. Thirty-four behind Japan and thirty-nine behind first place, Slovenia. Granted, these countries aren't just doing better than the U.S. on nutritional equality – they are also better at delivering healthcare to their residents. But healthcare is a topic for another book.

Let's set a bar for societal success to a level at which we can all find agreement. Healthy mommies are the best way to guarantee living, thriving babies. Maternal mortality rates give way to the infant mortality rates that continue to track all the babies who die in the first year of their lives. Globally, these deaths number in the millions. The U.S., at 40th place, has more than their share of these deaths.

Proper nutrition isn't just about living longer, it's about living more successfully. Malnutrition causes decreased cognitive ability in the children who survive starvation. Turns out, brain food isn't some old wives' tale. The human brain burns 25% of the calories needed to keep a human healthy – our bodies dedicate the other 75% of calories to respiration, locomotion, digestion, circulation, etc. You get the picture.

A culture or society that starves children literally debilitates their intellectual abilities, narrows society's future opportunities and diminishes the community's ability to thrive. Starving children hamstring a country's ability to flourish on the world stage.

Humans, with our disproportionately calorie-consumptive brains, have proven resourceful at both gathering and consuming nutrition. Where food is plentiful, our creativity knows no bounds. In times of plenty, harvesting, cooking and/or preparing meals have become integral parts of our celebrations.

Where sustenance is scarce, we've improvised to feed ourselves and our families. This book explores some of the ways the economically disadvantaged in the United States have scraped by – often creating family favorites conjured from otherwise-undesirable ingredients. As a seventy-something, rural Ohio gentleman told me when discussing his favorite breakfast – scrambled brains and eggs (made from beef brains his dad got for free from a local farmer) – "I had no idea it was disgusting. I thought it was delicious."

And no – this whole book isn't just a ghastly reminder that we can do better. Although we can. It's also sprinkled with recipes harvested from backyard gardens, foraged from roadsides and culled from humble, yet delectable sources.

Chapter One

It's All About Me

As a kid, we heard about hunger on a regular basis. What else should I have expected from an Irish Catholic mom but daily commentary about those who have nothing? I didn't get it as a kid – her obsession with hungry people. It was just a part of our lives. After all, it wasn't until my 39th year that I made it to Ireland – the land from whence my mom's family came. That's when I saw my first famine cemetery.

Have you seen one? A mass grave used to bury the hungry? It's not a cemetery in the sense that there's a patch of ground with tomb stones or markers. No, it's more a mound of earth where untold, nameless human remains clog the soil.

At first, my mind could not comprehend the scale of starvation that necessitates a mass grave. What sort of suffering does it represent? Not the tummy growling of one skipped meal. Nor the gnawing hunger of even a week of them. Not even the weakness or pain of a few months of deprivation. A famine cemetery indicates a whole community starving – starving to death. Young and old drained by prolonged malnourishment. And even though some family members sacrificed so others might eat, the whole group suffered from deficiencies so severe that entire clans perished.

My mom's clan came from that place. Her mom – my Nana – forced to leave home by scarcity, emigrated to the United States for two reasons. Firstly, they had extended family in America who told them that, in the U.S., fewer people went hungry. Secondly, back in Ireland after she left, fewer people would need to be fed. My Nana's departure improved the chances of survival for those who remained behind.

My grandmother never forgave her parents for sending her away. Nineteen and a new arrival to Boston, she stayed with a relation who had himself landed on ragged-soled feet across *the pond* from his home. He had room in his house for one more. I often wonder what that was like for her. How did he treat her? To my knowledge, she never told anyone about that part of her life. If she did, no one repeated the stories.

When life improved in Ireland, my Nana's parents sent for her. She ignored their letters. It seemed – as I ponder her reaction – that my grandmother would have preferred starvation to isolation and blamed her parents for not allowing her to make the choice for herself. She never went back. She never spoke to her mother again.

Hunger is cruel. It's hard to imagine how alone she felt. How rejected. So alone and rejected, in fact, that she found her forced expatriation even more horrible than starvation itself.

Nearly one hundred years later, I went back to Ireland in her place. I stared at the ground covering the mass graves, imagining what lay beneath the soil. I pictured the emaciated souls – some infants, others children, still more adults and elders – all interred before their time, for want of mere sustenance. I imagined my Nana there and understood why her parents forced her to leave for Boston.

My grandmother had much in common with the man I mentioned in the introduction. The man from Syria. Isolated from loved ones by the ravages of famine. Wondering if they're eating. Afraid to learn the truth. Feeling guilty about eating well.

It wasn't until I intellectually and physically connected with the conditions that drove my grandmother from the arms of her family – a family that loved her enough to send her away – that I understood my mother's obsession with feeding the poor. My mom, my Nana's daughter, took the mitigation of suffering and starvation around the world to be her own personal chore.

You see, my mom had not been raised by a woman who starved to death. She had been raised by a woman who lost her entire family to avoid starving.

In my mom's mind, caring about the hungry and feeding the poor achieved two important goals. While her actions might fill an empty belly. I think she wondered, perhaps, if her actions helped keep families together. Lessening hunger was my mom's way of respecting individuals, families, communities and the societies in which they thrived.

My mom, Genevieve, didn't feed every hungry person – but she fed a lot of them. When I was young, she rolled pennies for the Catholic Missions. Believing the missionaries brought food with their Bibles, she supported them until she left the church. When her awakened revulsion over sexism evolved and drove her from the Church of Rome, she supported non-denominational and secular charities. In the end, she sent money to world hunger programs like Oxfam and the Heifer Project. Look them up – they do great work.

Genevieve, born in 1926, faced her own hardships growing up. Living through the 20th century's Great Depression, my mom's Irish immigrant family resided in the marshlands outside Boston, Massachusetts. My grandmother raised poultry in the yard. Growing up, we heard stories of our Nana defending those chickens – with her bare hands when necessary – from beasts that wandered the marshes in search of prey. Living in the 1930's Depression era in the U.S. may have been easier than surviving turn-of-the-century famine in Ireland, but only by degree.

Life in America was easier, but not easy. My mom remembered hunger, privation, need. My uncle Buddy, Genevieve's eldest brother, died of tuberculosis.

When she could, my grandmother and those of her generation and cultural background, worked as servants in the homes of others. Life was hard.

As a kid, I adored my Nana. I never thought of her as a woman who had suffered. She showed no signs of abuse. She worshipped me and I felt it. My mom did the same. My Aunt Rita would joke that Genevieve was the only woman she'd ever met who had five only children. Each of us was *spoiled rotten* with warmth and security – as if such gifts could actually cause a child to *spoil* – to *go bad*.

Spending time around strong women who showered others with

affection made it easy for us – me and my four siblings – to admire their ideals. I guess that's why I, too, grew up pre-occupied by the plight of those less fortunate. Privately, I've helped when and how I could. Professionally, I've gravitated to jobs that brought me nearer to folks experiencing what I can only imagine my Nana lived through as a child and young mom.

In the beginning of my career, as a member of the media, I witnessed and related stories of folks in distress. Later, as a shelter worker, I became intimately aware of how individuals and families struggle to survive.

Witnessing suffering is like watching human fireworks. So much is going off at once that you miss the details while staring at the bigger picture. At first, working directly with the unhoused, I concentrated on housing. Then, more than a decade ago, I began observing more closely the impressive way people struggled to feed themselves and their families. Whenever possible, they didn't just get food – they made a meal. Distinctly different activities! Staving off hunger lacks the ceremony and solemnity associated with preparing and experiencing a meal.

Even Laura Ingalls Wilder – in her books about frontier life in the nineteenth century – told tales of starvation that included the ritual of grinding wheat in the family's old coffee mill. Her mom would then bake the *bread*, and the entire family came together to share it.

After years working with those experiencing homelessness, it became quite apparent that being unhoused is only one aspect of poverty. People packed forty or fifty to a shelter, sharing one kitchen, exhibit different coping mechanisms in all aspects of life. Without privacy, the unhoused struggle in plain sight. This book is a result of my observations fueled by my natural curiosity about my own family's struggle to provide.

In today's parlance, my Nana experienced homelessness. She came to the U.S. and doubled up with another family. Doubled up is a term used by some members of the housing community to describe folks who live with each other when rooflessness would be their only other option. Lack of housing is a visible sign of poverty. Hunger is another, often less visible, indicator.

Hungry enough to leave Ireland, it's likely my grandmother arrived in the U.S., hungry as well. Documents detailing steerage passage cite limited amounts of food. And, odds are, she was hungry when she got off the boat.

For decades, I've written about homelessness. I've tried to translate the cultural differences that come from having nowhere to go. No place of one's own.

Then, about five years ago, it occurred to me that if I told readers what I've witnessed about how folks eat, society might better understand that it's a herculean task to make ends meet. And, sadly, it's timely, because what my Nana experienced a century ago is still required of millions of Americans struggling to survive today.

Nana Mary's *Fight a Fox for Your Chicken* Turkey Soup

This is based on a story that went through our family. One night my Nana ran out into the yard, butcher knife in hand, to protect her chickens from a fox that had gotten in their pen. Bloody and triumphant, my Nana fended off the fox but was forced to butcher a mortally wounded chicken.

Everyone loved her turkey soup which – customarily – was not made with chicken. Although I have no doubt that all the soups she made had at least some chicken fat in them.

- Turkey scraps and bones (save the skin after discarding the bones, etc.)
- Leftover turkey
- Salt
- Black pepper
- Vegetables – especially celery, onions, carrots
- Rice
- Fat for sautéing vegetables (could be saved chicken fat or bacon grease from prior meals. You might use butter if you're rich or have a cow).

I have to believe there were three secrets to this nearly perfect soup. One is that the bones and other scraps were boiled until they disintegrated and literally thickened the water as it became broth. Secondly, don't make this soup unless you have hours of prep time. Lastly, using a strainer to remove the remnants that haven't dissolved from boiling is advised. This is your turkey stock. Discard bones. Save the skin.

Sauté extremely finely chopped vegetables. That's the second secret. Chop the veggies into tiny pieces. Shredding the celery and onion would work fine. Chop the carrots a bit (not much) larger. Add the turkey, skin and turkey stock.

Add *some* salt and pepper. *Some* salt and *some* pepper are literally the right amount to make it taste yummy. *Some* salt is not the same as *some* sugar that, for example, you might add to a cup of tea. *Some* always meant the right amount. Good luck. (Obviously you might start with what could be *less than some* and add until you get the *correct some*, but that will be a process).

About a half hour before you intend to serve the soup, add some rice. (See above – obviously *some* rice depends on how much stock you have). My Nana's soup was always soup-like, never stew-like. So don't use too much rice or you'll need to add water and then you'll dilute the flavor.

When Things Got Better, She Made These Biscuits to Go with Her Turkey Soup

I have no idea what it was like for Genevieve when she was little. I am unaware if they would have these biscuits with soup when she was young. They had so little during the Depression. I doubt that they had turkey then, either – just the chickens from the yard if they stopped laying or were born male. These biscuits – as she called them – were, in reality, the most delicious yeast rolls I've ever eaten. No one in our large, extended family has ever made them so good since my Nana died in 1967. But this is the recipe as recounted down through the years and reconstructed by my sister, Claire.

Claire described the difference between our grandmother's yeast rolls and anyone else's, "What Nana would do is just get butter all over her fingers so the dough wouldn't stick. And all that extra butter made the difference."

- 2-1/4 teaspoons dry yeast
- 1/4 cup warm water
- 2 to 2-1/2 cups flour
- 2 tablespoons sugar
- 1/2 teaspoon salt
- 1/2 cup milk
- ½ cup butter (or more)

Soften yeast in 1/4 cup warm water in a large mixing bowl. Let stand 5 minutes. Add 1 cup flour, sugar, salt, milk and butter. Mix well by hand. Add 1 cup flour and, again, mix well. Continue adding in enough additional flour (if needed) to make a soft dough.

Turn dough on lightly floured surface and knead 2 to 3 minutes. Place dough in a buttered bowl, turning once to coat. Cover and let rise in a warm, draft-free place for 30 minutes or more, until doubled.

Knead well and divide dough into 12 equal pieces. Shape into balls. Place in greased 8-inch round pan. Our grandmother often rolled them with lots of butter into more of a crescent pattern. Rolling them up that way got butter chunks mixed through the dough. If using this method, place them on a cookie sheet.

Let rise 30 minutes or more, until doubled. You can let rolls rise in a closed oven with a bowl you filled with boiling water on a rack beneath them.

Preheat oven to 375°F. Bake rolls for 20 to 25 minutes, or until done. Tapping on top of rolls, they should sound hollow. Remove from pan. Serve warm.

My mom made variations of fishy delicacies from her family's native island of Ireland that – for a time in the Boston area – could be had inexpensively. Irish Catholics had an added burden (as does everyone with dietary rules dictated by religion or digestive disorders) of having to eat certain foods at certain times. Genevieve fed a family of seven with fish every Friday night. Luckily, in those days, canned fish could be had affordably. Who knows what would have become of our mortal souls if we'd eaten bologna or hot dogs.

When my brothers and sisters and I were young and resources were scarce, she made creamed canned tuna on toast. My sister Marian swears up and down that she loved it. She recently told me that she couldn't wait to get home from school on Friday afternoon because it was creamed tuna night. Not me.

And for toast? We ate a lot of generic white bread. I don't think the kind of thin pasty white bread we ate is even available for sale anymore. The bread, more air than flour, squished down incredibly well and could be formed into other shapes – then stay that way! My favorite smashing-the-cheap-white-bread activity consisted of pretending to serve each other communion like we saw at church on Sundays. We would unscrew the metal cap from the glass saltshaker and press out wafers from the bread. So much for our mortal souls, but it was great fun.

It wasn't always creamed tuna on toast. We'd also have frozen fish sticks (I smothered them in ketchup) and, on special occasions, she made creamed canned salmon on toast. These two creamed fish recipes are identical. Just swap out salmon for tuna as desired.

Genevieve's Creamed Tuna on Toast

- 3 tablespoons fat
- 3 tablespoons flour
- 1 can tuna
- 2 cups milk
- Black pepper to taste
- Half a loaf of ghastly white bread

Melt the fat – no lard or chicken fat if avoiding meat. Butter, margarine – even cooking oil works. Once liquified in a saucepan, add the flour. Mix to create a paste. Add milk and keep stirring, ideally with a whisk or a fork. Dump in contents of tuna can (drained or not). Toast the bread and spoon the mixture onto two side-by-side slices of the toast. Pepper to taste. The canned nature of the tuna makes it a bit salty already. If desired, follow the same recipe but use salmon.

Less frequently, Genevieve made the world's best fish chowder. In honor of John F. Kennedy, a man she danced with in a club on Cape Cod one evening before either of them was married. I've put her recipe for fish chowder in the chapter on food stamps. Fish chowder is rumored to have been Kennedy's favorite meal. And because he's the president who inaugurated the United States Department of Agriculture feeding program for the underprivileged in our country, I think it's only fair one of Genevieve's signature dishes be found in that chapter.

The delicacy I will reward you with here is Genevieve's baked stuffed lobster. For hundreds of years coastal residents throughout New England feasted on what others considered "the trash of the sea."

At one time, lobsters were so plentiful, so unwanted and, consequently, so cheap, that the state of Maine fed them morning, noon and night to the inmates of the Maine State Penitentiary. The result? Prison lobster riots. The Island Institute has documented similar riots against the glut of cheap salmon served in so-called poor houses and jails. I'll leave links in the bibliography if you want to learn more.

Genevieve's Baked Stuffed Lobster

- Same number of lobsters as people you intend to feed
- Scallops
- Butter - melted
- Ritz crackers - crushed
- Garlic powder

No other seasoning necessary – remember, the crackers are salty
Take freshly sliced and gutted lobster (remove tomalley, etc.).
Combine melted butter with garlic. This is purely a matter of taste and quantities depend on the number of people you're feeding. For four lobsters, use one pound of butter and a half teaspoon of garlic powder. Fold in crushed Ritz crackers.

My tireless editor, Cheryl Dunn Bychek wanted to know how many crackers. I polled the sisters – we can't remember. But I would say the better part of a long sleeve that comes out of the Ritz box. Less one or two we'd snatch when she'd turn her back to work on the meal.

For four lobsters, twelve large scallops will do nicely. Cut the scallops in half or quarters, depending on personal preference. Stuff them into the split opening in the lobsters and pack the openings around them with the Ritz/butter/garlic concoction. Remaining cracker mixture goes over the top. Bake in a pre-heated 400-degree oven for 15 to 20 minutes.

You may know that lobsters should not be eaten if they die more than a few minutes before you cook them. My mom couldn't tolerate the idea of boiling the creatures alive, so when she boiled or steamed lobster, she'd have my dad conk them on the back of the head with a hammer before throwing them in the pot. In the case of this dish, she'd have someone else use a large carving knife to slice them down the middle (often my father, but she was grateful to anyone in the vicinity who would take the task off her hands). Be prepared to stuff the lobsters with the scallops and cracker mixture as soon as the dastardly deed is done.

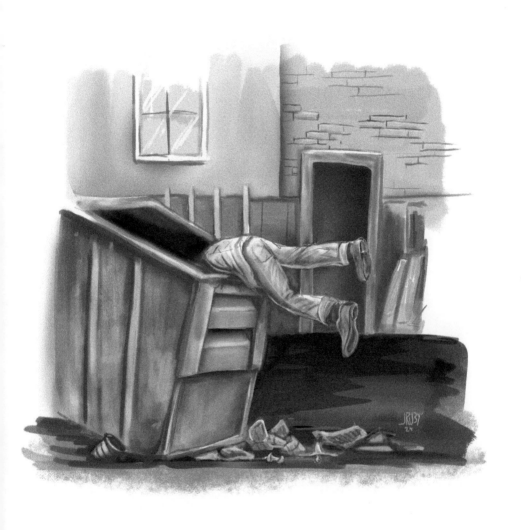

How the Other Half Lives

Chapter Two
Us

Late one afternoon, I sat at my desk in a central Pennsylvania emergency shelter. As the light outside my window changed, aromas made their way down the hall. I glanced at the time on the computer screen: 5:15. The shelter guests had started cooking their dinners.

We called them guests in those days. Early in the founding of the emergency shelter agency where I worked, they'd decided that guest sounded nicer than client. Hoping to make people feel invited instead of desperate – the misnomer stuck. Folks in search of warmth, safety, security, a mailing address, respite, or help navigating our nation's convoluted housing system filtered in our door each day. In all the years I worked there, I remember only two days when we weren't filled to capacity. Otherwise, we turned people away for lack of space.

At first, the shelter's *guests* were single men and women. After a few years, the need for family shelter became so apparent that policies changed. The facilities got no more kid-friendly, but the kids needed housing, so *guests* they became. The smoking area, our only outdoor recreation area, became a makeshift playground. No swings or slides, but more than enough exhausted adults, smoldering cigarette butts and secondhand smoke.

I've worked for a few front-line housing agencies. Some provided transitional and permanent housing. Two provided emergency housing with private rooms. On the night the aromas stirred my imagination, my employer offered only the most rudimentary assistance to an unhoused population as varied as society at large.

For years I worked from an office in a resource center, where our communal kitchen had two refrigerators, one stove, a sink and a dishwasher. Each night there'd be a flurry of activity as people prepared meals for themselves and their families. Afterward, the *guests* would leave – journeying to local church where they would sleep on the floor.

With rare exception, we never got any rich people through our shelter doors. Oh sure, every now and again, our agency would clear out the unhoused and host an *open house* for the community. A few visiting dignitaries or donors would stop over. The *guests*, removed under the auspices of protecting confidentiality, scampered off to the library or a nearby park.

I dunno for sure, but if I moved you out of your residence and snooped around when you were gone, I think you might feel like your privacy had been invaded. Despite the inconvenience and invasiveness, I don't remember those events ever yielding many donations. Seldom were the visitors wealthy enough – or so moved to generosity – that it made much of a difference. I think the real reason my boss led tours of the resource center was to keep the NIMBY (not in my back yard) folks in check. "Nothing to see here, boys and girls. You can move along and quit worrying now."

Sadly, keeping NIMBYs at bay proved imperative over the years, as people who had something more and someplace to keep it resented those who had nothing. As the resentment festers, there persists a long-term low-grade effort to keep "those people" out of the neighborhood.

The super-rich never came for the tours. The moneyed class doesn't seem to have homeless shelters on their radar. For the most part, the wealthier segments of society have all managed to steer clear.

Not knowing.

Not wanting to know.

Or perhaps just thinking they already know more than their wealthy selves need to know. Those people – them – the folks experiencing homelessness – they get what they deserve.

It's incumbent on me to say this – nobody deserves homelessness. If people took a closer look, they'd see that. Homelessness is a byproduct of inequity. It isn't caused by the three stereotypical scapegoats – drugs or alcohol or mental illness. Plenty of folks experiencing those realities do so from the comfort of their homes. Plenty of rich folks share those unfortunate conditions and it doesn't make them homeless.

That's because homelessness is about poverty. Period!

No one with the means to do otherwise would go to a shelter. Ever. Nearly everyone with resources isn't even curious. We could open the shelters to outsiders a thousand times a day, and the community at large – especially those who need to know what shelters are like, wouldn't bother.

It's not just the comfortable who lack insight – it's the powerful as well. Someone should tell the U.S. Department of Housing and Urban Development (HUD) what the rest of us, working on the ground level, understand. Nobody lives in a shelter if they have even a remote chance of living elsewhere.

A few years back, HUD changed their regulations. Used to be that you could show up at a shelter and get help. Now, HUD requires people seeking shelter prove their homelessness in order to get assistance from government-funded shelters. The implication there? That folks with adequate homes would choose to stay in a shelter instead. I'd laugh out loud right now if it weren't so tragic. Requiring folks to prove homelessness is an indication of how disconnected lawmakers and administrators are from the needs of their constituents.

By the time I started working at that beleaguered emergency facility with the one kitchen and the folks tramping off to sleep on church floors, we sheltered pretty much everyone who wasn't on a child sex offender registry. Even people with prior violent history were our *guests*. We literally hosted rape victim guests within yards of rapist *guests* – all together – on the borrowed floor of a nearby church.

Shortly after the population changed from single adults to everybody, so did the daytime experience. At its inception, the church-sponsored outreach mirrored hundreds of other overnight shelters across the nation.

Early on, people experiencing homelessness learned about the shelter by word of mouth. The story spread rapidly through the housing-insecure community to other folks in need of shelter. Folks would learn which of the churches was open to them each month. Every night, dozens of displaced guys and gals would knock at the church door and ask to stay. Volunteers stayed with them at night and offered what they could for well-meaning advice.

By the time I became Operations Manager, my boss had worked with the community and built a resource center. The building had showers, hand-me-down junior high lockers donated by a local school department, a storage closet filled with donated goods and a kitchen.

The feds love numbers – especially low numbers. Wildly incorrect numbers are collected, by design. See my book *Still Left Out in America* for how the HUD PIT count works – or doesn't.

At any rate, I kept my own accounting of our census. I met thousands of people and in my years and about 55 percent of them had incomes. Some were elderly or disabled, others had low-wage jobs paying way too little for a person to have a home. Employers that paid less than a living wage managed to keep many of their employees because our nation's shelter networks subsidize their greed. Companies without consciences needn't pay a living wage if a shelter nearby will support the workforce with showers and a church floor.

Our society operates based on the foolhardy premise that the "Feed a Man a Fish" dilemma is real. You know, "Do you give a man a fish or teach him to fish?"

Obviously, if you want the community to thrive, you do both. Feed him until he's capable of feeding himself. With multinational corporations, the question is a little murkier. More like this: If companies don't pay folks enough to live, do you give them shelter until the company's policy improves? Or do you deny shelter to individuals employed by corporations that should pay better – further punishing their workforce and starving the company of employees, until they choose to improve wages and benefits so the workforce can afford to live in dignity?

Ah, America!

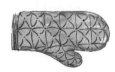

Back to my personal, anecdotal statistics. In the better part of ten years, I personally had contact with thousands of folks in need of housing – 55 percent of whom had an income and 30 percent more who were their children. A full 85 percent of the folks I sheltered were the working poor and their kids. And those kids needed to eat!

Where was I? Oh yeah. It was 5:15 p.m. and smells wafted down the hall to my office. My stomach growled. But – I had a rule, and I never broke it. No matter how good something smelled, I never ate any of it. Sure, there were some concoctions our guests created that I really wanted to taste. But, I had a fridge at home. Hell, I had a home!

Rejecting an offer of food can hurt the feelings of those who are offering. Food is a gesture of goodwill, a cultural exchange, a common experience where like-minded friends or colleagues can meet. Cooking is a love language, a statement of concern, a form of welcoming and a wonderful way to express gratitude. But, still, I promised myself I would never eat food prepared by someone experiencing food insecurity – unless I paid for it.

Often, I would walk into a situation where a person preparing a succulent-smelling meal offered to share. I invariably feigned fullness to avoid taking a portion of what they'd prepared – hoping my stomach wouldn't growl and catch me in my lie. If I really wanted to try it, I had a standard offer, "I'll buy groceries next week if you'll make it for me then." Sometimes I'd suggest that I purchase the ingredients so they could teach me to make the delicious-looking and/or -smelling concoction. Feed a Pat a meal? No, teach her to make her own!

That one night, as I wandered down the hallway – like a cartoon Bugs Bunny following the scent of carrots – I stumbled over a few new toddlers. One of my colleagues had performed an intake that nearly doubled our pre-school numbers. I approached the stove, introducing myself to a young mom stirring an enormous pot of sauce. "Hi, I'm Pat. Came out here to see who'd improved the smell of the place!" I announced.

"I'm Christy. Sorry about the rug rats." (Ironically there was no rug. Just a constantly filthy floor despite its nightly washings).

"No trouble at all. Just make sure you keep them in your line of sight. One of my colleagues might have told you, but we can't guarantee their safety. You must keep them with you, even if you go to the restroom."

Christy nodded.

"Easier said than done, I agree." I continued, "If you smoke cigarettes, you need to take them to the smoking area. You get it?"

Christy, wide-eyed, nodded again. I thought I might've come on a little strong. Point made. I changed the subject. "Whatcha cooking?"

"The sheriff put us out of our home. Our septic blew, and the landlord won't fix it. I grabbed everything I had in the freezer and browned it in this pot with a few jars of tomato sauce."

I smiled, "Smells good. There's lots of dry pasta in the storeroom if you need it."

We always had lots of donated pasta.

Christy smiled again. I thought, *she's remarkably composed considering all she's been through.*

As though she'd read my mind, she spoke again, "It makes me feel better to cook."

I looked around the common area. There weren't too many folks seated at the tables because the soup kitchen up the road fed folks at 4:30 each afternoon leaving behind only a few individuals too incapacitated to walk a half mile for a meal.

"I figured I'd share what we have with these folks." Christy gestured to the other guests assembled at the tables. "If they're going to have to put up with my little ones, least I can do is feed them."

Ahhh, I thought. *Food working its magic – making Christy feel comfortable while it served as a bribe to a few handicapped and elderly folks who might make better allies than adversaries.*

"Make sure you label any leftovers before you put them in the fridge. Anything unlabeled is fair game. Even marked, sometimes people will eat your food." I smiled down at the three-year-old hugging her mom's leg, "Put the date on it, too. We have a facilities manager with a penchant for throwing out unmarked food."

Christy struggled to keep smiling as fear, shock, and unknowing took over her face. "We've never had to do this before," she offered – almost as an excuse for why nothing I said ever occurred to her before she, too, became homeless. Her face flushed as she told me, "We'll try to get out as soon as we can." She meant it, too.

She had a truck to unpack – the one her husband had parked in front of the shelter – a U-Haul they'd hurriedly filled before the sheriff permanently locked the door. Even more urgent – they had left a family member behind. Their dog remained tied on his lead at the house. They had plans to go back in the morning and feed him.

"I know this is tough." I commiserated with the young mom. "My job is to meet people on the toughest day of their lives. I'm sorry to say this is it. Today is yours and still you're here feeding others." A tear rolled down her cheek as I spoke.

"Let me know if you need anything." I offered that platitude as I did every day, all day. Even though what she needed was a home. And, on that matter, I was no help at all.

I'd like to say Christy and her adorable family left the next day. Happy endings happen, but never that fast. Instead, and eventually, she and her husband rented a storage unit, returning the U-Haul, horribly overdue. We got their dog registered as a service animal to assist with their autistic child and the pooch became a welcome additional guest at the shelter. After more than a year, the family moved on – becoming what they are now – stably and permanently housed.

I ran into Christy and her daughter in Lincoln Memorial Park, a few years later. We chatted while local artist and civic activist Jim Griffith kneeled on the ground. With bright red and yellow paint, he stenciled the sidewalk with the names of people buried under the grass nearby. A few decades earlier, urban renewal advocates convinced Carlisle, Pennsylvania to eliminate one of the Black cemeteries in that history-drenched town. A half hour up the road from Gettysburg National Cemetery, where President Lincoln *could not dedicate, could not consecrate, could not hallow the ground*, public officials removed the gravestones, but left the bodily remains interred. Over an entire community's Black antecedents, the white borough council built a small park.

Rather than allow their loved ones to be lost to posterity, a local woman scoured more than a hundred years of newspaper burial notices and reconstructed a list of the people whose memorials were deliberately expunged.

Christy's youngest approached Jim and asked, "Why are you painting those names?"

He explained what happened. Told her that the names represented the people buried under the park. Confused the youngster asked, "If they took away the stones, how will you know where to leave flowers?"

How indeed?

Christy's World and Two Recipes She Uses to Feed an Army

I took the opportunity, once I met up with Christy again, to ask how things had changed since she'd become stably housed. She shared some recent stories with me. She explained that her kids liked their new home but still had trouble playing outside. Quiet kids, they preferred to keep to themselves. After the year-plus they spent being shushed and scolded if they ran and played, it's hard to tell if their silence and solitude aren't just residue of a life surrounded by an ever-changing cast of hundreds.

Christy never complains. She's more grateful than her circumstances call for – her gratitude gives her perspective that makes her graceful and calm. We chatted about her new life. Having her own place and things getting back to "normal." Ending homelessness doesn't return someone to the life they had before they lost their housing. Homelessness changes a person. Christy's stably housed, but she's different.

Still, now that she has a kitchen of her own, she makes dishes that remind her of days when she'd feed everyone in sight. The following is our brief exchange about cooking – as well as some recipes or tips for feeding the masses.

Me: How'd you get along after you left the shelter?

Christy: For years and years, we survived on $70 for groceries every two weeks. Whatever was on sale at the grocery store, that's what we'd eat. Every now and then they'd have buy-one-get-one-free specials. Those helped. I felt so fortunate when I could get two pot roasts!

Everything we bought had to stretch for four meals. A whole chicken or a pot roast. I'd make recipes handed down through the years. If I could get the ingredients I'd make Ham, Rice and Eggs because it made so ridiculously much food.

Me: Things are better now?

Christy: Oh yes. It's still a struggle because my kids developed food allergies or intolerances. We couldn't just go to a soup kitchen or pick up donations at the food bank because one daughter has a gluten intolerance, and another can't have dairy. You probably know that the first thing food banks want to give you is a loaf of bread and a gallon of milk. I felt like such an asshole. I mean who goes into a food bank and turns food away?

Me: There are not a lot of vegetables in your recipes.

Christy: It's very difficult to get veggies. If they're fresh you absolutely cannot afford organic. If you do manage to get some fresh produce, you have to worry about your investment. Did you spend your money wisely? What if it goes bad before the kids eat it? When will it spoil? And if it's fruit – your investment is completely wiped out in a couple of days. You think the money will last a week, but you buy fruit and it's gone in two days.

Me: I remember that time our shelter was at First United Church of Christ and a donor had purchased cereal, milk and dozens of bananas. Do you remember that?

Christy: No, I don't think we were there then.

Me: The guests were overjoyed. But I hear what you're saying about the investment. The bananas had all been eaten within minutes.

Ham, Rice and Eggs

- A ham steak or ham hocks
- Rice
- A dozen eggs
- Fat

"Cook off the ham (boil). Pick off meat and/or chop it up. Put the ham in the water with the uncooked rice. Cooking with the ham increases the flavor of the rice. Even if you don't have a lot of ham, the rice absorbs the flavor. Cook the rice. As much of it as you can. Two, three, four cups doesn't matter – the more people, the more rice you need to make. Put the fat in the pan and scramble the eggs and add to ham and rice. It feeds a small army for $5.00."

That price estimate has likely gone up a bit since Christy and I last spoke.

Lipton Soup Gravy

- Lipton soup mix. (The extra noodle kind if they have it).
- Corn starch
- Rice
- Any leftover meat of any kind – if you have it.
- Chinese chow mein noodles

"Make the Lipton soup. Use cornstarch to thicken it. Add meat if you have some. Prepare the rice and pour the thickened soup gravy on top.

Top with chow mein noodles if you have them – they make the meal crunchy and fancy!"

Chapter Three

Shelter Improv

When I first considered the title, *Humble Pie*, I toyed with calling this book *Eating Crow*. If you keep reading, later in this book you'll find I titled a chapter that way, instead. But for the book, it struck me that I witnessed far more humility than humiliation. *Eating Crow* conveys a message that someone's been knowingly disgraced. It implies a disgruntled acceptance by the economically disadvantaged in the way they're forced to sustain themselves.

But that's not the case. However, the marginalized managed to feed themselves – from what I could tell – they rarely questioned why their end of the stick came up so short. I can't remember even a handful of individuals who complained about their food or even their unnecessarily arduous situations, for that matter. To the contrary, in fact. For all the suffering I've witnessed, I generally witnessed gratitude – even for situations or meals that neither you nor I might find palatable.

Homeless shelters are human dumpsters. All across the United States, the poor, the tired, the huddled masses collect at their doorsteps. Often, when hopelessly unhoused people search desperately for help, they're referred to one organization or another. Commonly, an ambulance or police officer will dump human beings at shelters without waiting to hear if the agency has available space. The public servant drives off – as the human dumpster overflows.

I remember one night a park ranger from Maryland drove to our Pennsylvania emergency shelter because he'd found a woman camping, without authorization, along the Appalachian Trail. A few days earlier, her apartment building had burned to the ground. The displaced tenant had no renters' insurance. She'd lost everything.

Folks who present this way – with nothing (a nothing most folks can't imagine) – need clothing, toiletries, prescription medication refills, vital documents, food. Our shelter had a small pantry of donated non-perishables.

Standard operating procedure for folks experiencing homelessness included background checks, a trip to the police station and lots of paperwork. Why the police station? We sent folks there in case the cops had a warrant for their arrest. Folks who did, didn't come back. Perhaps they were arrested, but more likely they just walked away from our shelter and never checked in with the police at all. Either way, they never came back.

The United States does have a limited number of zero-barrier shelters. In places such as these, folks can walk in and get help: no background check, no ID, no problem. I tried to open one in our town. Pre-pandemic. A local church agreed to let us use their common area for some no-questions-asked mass sheltering on frigid nights. Then COVID-19 struck. Mass sheltering became deadly. Other organizers revamped the concept, removing the zero-barrier part. They made it a cold-weather shelter instead, shifting housing street people from a church common area to the motels emptied by the pandemic. Because the new concept involved for-profit businesses, we were unable to convince the community leaders that we didn't need background checks for the people we served. *Too much liability.*

Let's talk liability. For individuals fleeing violence, revealing one's identity seems riskier than freezing-cold temperatures. Sadly, the excuses by the authorities are always a variation on the rule. "We can't just help *anyone*… Hotel insurance companies demand identification."

Etcetera, etcetera, etcetera… In the meantime, people freeze or starve on the street. Or they freeze or burn to death in their homes.

Too often, when the fuel runs out and desperate folks employ unsafe heating practices, they can asphyxiate in their sleep or light their surroundings on fire. I'll put a few links to such tragedies in the bibliography – if you're curious.

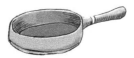

One cold, winter night, a 37-year-old, poorly dressed woman appeared at the shelter door. Frightened and alone, she asked if we had a place for her to stay. I'll call her Stephanie. Stephanie needed a shower, warm clothes, food and safety. After I finished her paperwork and created a paper ID for her – she had none of her own – she picked through our donation pile and found some clean clothes. We gave her shampoo, soap, a toothbrush and some tampons.

Fifteen minutes later, she returned to my office. Clean, with her new clothes hanging from her tiny frame, she looked and seemed much better. She wore socks but hadn't yet put on her shoes. I asked if she needed shoes. If she'd been unable to find any in the donation bin. She shook her head, No.

She explained that she'd slept outside several nights in a row and her feet had frozen. It hurt to put on her shoes. I asked her to show me. She wouldn't. I offered to call her an ambulance. She declined.

Over the years, a nurse friend of mine has made shelter calls when tough-to-cajole folks needed medical care. I offered to call Tracey. Stephanie said, "No." She explained that her family was looking for her. They were rich. They'd hired private detectives. She couldn't go a hospital because they'd find her. I had no idea if any of her story was true. I couldn't force her to get help. I could let her stay, or I could make her leave. Those were my only options. Of course, I let her stay.

Warm and clean, she walked in her stocking feet with me. We went to the storage closet, and she found all we had to offer. Cases of ramen noodles. Cases of brand name and no name macaroni and cheese. Canned spaghetti products. Canned vegetables.

I showed her the common area of the resource center, where the shelter had just those two refrigerators for the fifty or so occupants to share. Folks who stayed in the shelter purchased and stored perishables in the public fridges. All the food inside them was privately owned.

I explained the system to Stephanie. I offered to ask the group if anyone had some milk to share. Frightened, Stephanie didn't like that idea.

I know what you're wondering. Why didn't the shelter have a refrigerator with perishables donated that everyone could share? I wondered the same thing. At first, I was told we didn't have room for another fridge. After a year or so of badgering, I convinced the director to let me get an extra and stock it with milk, juice, eggs and butter. I left shortly after that. I have no idea if it's still there.

Anyway, that night, I watched Stephanie move slowly on her sore feet. Using what she found in the storage room, she made herself some dinner.

Stephanie's Humble Attempt at Healthy

- One large can mixed vegetables
- One package generic macaroni with powered cheese product

Empty contents of mixed vegetables into a saucepan. Place on stove over medium high heat. Do not add additional water. Add the macaroni product from the package – reserving the cheese powder for later. Bring vegetables and pasta to a boil. When pasta is cooked thoroughly, add nearly the entire contents of cheese packet. The remaining moisture from the vegetables will help dissolve the powdered cheese. Or plate the vegetable and pasta mixture and sprinkle with remaining cheese powder.

Stephanie evidenced some pretty severe symptoms of mental illness. She did not pose an immediate threat to herself or anyone else. She preferred to be left alone. Still, some nights, she would cry out in her sleep. Some of the residents found it unnerving but she stayed off by herself and the other guests gave her a wide berth. I liked her a lot. At quiet moments she would visit with me in my office. Very bright, we'd talk about science, animals and other things that interested her.

In the few weeks she stayed with us, her feet got worse. She became more frightened. She asked me to find her family on Facebook so she could see them. I did. She made me promise not to contact them. I told her I wouldn't and I never did.

One of the other employees at the shelter didn't like Stephanie. One night, unbeknownst to me, she evicted her from the shelter for yelling in her sleep. The employee said she couldn't reconcile having a person like that around the little children who slept at the shelter. "Those kids needed their sleep." Fair enough – if the world were fair. But this is 21st century U.S. suburban homelessness – newborn to ninety – there ain't nothing fair about it.

Some of the other unhoused folks told me they saw her sleeping in the bushes outside the church after she'd been expelled. I tried to find her. I failed. For weeks I kept trying. I kept failing.

Cooking = Nurturing
Even in a Shelter

Back in '09, I took over as VP of a transitional shelter. We housed people in an historic downtown hotel. A nice old building with good bones and regular upkeep. This shelter was one of the few decent places to land – in the entire country – if you found yourself unhoused. Across the hall from my office, a little old woman from Pittsburgh lived in a small room with a private bath, a dorm-sized fridge, a toaster oven and her husband's ashes in a cardboard box on the windowsill.

Friendly and welcoming, Louise and I often chatted in our doorways. The most remarkable smells floating from her room. It is with great horror that I recount that she cooked everything in that toaster oven of hers! Including friend chicken! (BTW, Louise made the best fried chicken I've ever had).

Here's what I remember of her recipe. I found a similar one online by a chef named, CJ. His blog url is in the bibliography. I think if you try his recipe, using normal frying techniques, you won't be disappointed.

Taste-of-Home Fried Chicken

- Bone in chicken parts, skin on
- *I bought her thighs when she made it for me – delish!*
- Milk
- Spices (including salt and pepper)
- Flour
- Baking powder
- Corn starch
- Cooking oil

There are no amounts for any of this. Sorry. Wash chicken parts and dry with clean paper towel. Add spices to the milk. Pierce the skin and the meat of the chicken, lightly, with a fork. Don't make too many holes, and not too big. Soak the meat in the milk mixture for about an hour. Mix dry ingredients. When you put the chicken into the flour mixture, be sure to push it in good. So it really sticks.

(I can't believe I'm about to type this). Take the shallow baking pan of your toaster oven and fill it almost to the lip with cooking oil. Close the oven and turn it on high until the oil gets hot – but not too hot! Place a few pieces of chicken in the hot oil and fry. Don't close the door. Turn chicken and do this expertly until the chicken is perfectly golden and cooked through. DO NOT DO THIS, EVER!

I really only included this recipe because fried chicken was Louise's comfort food, her love language. Preparing it and eating it sustained her the way breathing did – maybe more so. Homelessness doesn't mean you lose your past, your culture, your comfort. Homelessness means that keeping those basic human needs alive means risk. And Louise risked burning the shelter to the ground for a simple taste of home.

Taci's Chili Bake

Taci had two kids and a hubby. Except the hubby got diagnosed with a terminal illness. By the time Taci and the girls came to the shelter, the couple had decided to divorce so that Chad could get the Medicaid assistance he needed to survive. Taci worked full time at a warehouse overnights, allowing her to care for the girls by day. Taci made her chili bake regularly for the kids because they loved it. They still do. Taci smiled when she told me that occasionally she'll whip up this comfort food that harkens back from a time when they had very little comfort.

- One can Hormel Chili (you can use off brand if it's all you have)
- One package generic macaroni with powered cheese product

Boil macaroni noodles as directed on the box. Drain. Heat chili and layer over the noodles. Sprinkle the chili and noodles with cheese powder from the packet included in the dinner.

I love the way Taci raised her kids. They're both in high school now and they're great people. I remember each night seeing those kids do their homework surrounded by strangers. I remember mornings watching the children get up from the floor of the church and pack their rolling suitcases to leave. They would walk down the street at 6:30 a.m. dragging their belongings behind them. A stranger might have unwittingly guessed that the children were headed off on vacation. Of course, that stranger would've been wrong.

Eventually, Taci remarried. She, her new husband and the girls got a home not far from the one Chad had gotten earlier in their story. Chad keeps fighting for his life. The girls see him every day.

Max's Dollar Store Potluck
Homeless Homemade Holiday Fare

Max experienced homelessness on several occasions. An adult orphan, with no family to rely on, Max battled with mental illness and would periodically get evicted. A talented artist and IT specialist, Max worked even though he had no home. Losing one's housing due to eviction generally includes losing security deposits and getting bad references. It's not that a person with bad references can't get a new apartment. They can, if they have enough money to guarantee many months of security instead of just one. Max would get evicted, experience homelessness, then spend the better part of a year saving the money needed to get a new apartment.

Max has since broken that cycle. But a decade or so ago, Max languished in a better-than-most emergency shelter. Each resident had a single room with a door that locked. They shared a bathroom and kitchen. During that time, his workplace planned a Christmas party and asked all the employees to bring something homemade. This was what he made.

Please note – Dollar stores generally sell in very small amounts. Because – well – dollar. And a dollar won't buy much. Purchasing in those small dollar-increments, Max could make cheesy pepperoni bread, enough to bring to his small office party, for about fifteen dollars.

- Dollar store bread dough mix
- Dollar store sausage (pepperoni if you can find it)
- Dollar store cheese

Mix bread dough according to directions on package (add water and mix). Pat between your hands or roll out on counter. If you don't have a rolling pin, a water bottle works well. Layer cheese and pepperoni on bread. Bake according to instructions on the package. For holiday parties, shape the bread into wreaths, stockings, trees, shamrocks, eggs, etc.

Max recommends adding fresh vegetables or a sauce (sometimes a nice alfredo sauce) if you're not too poor. But if you are too poor, the folks at work will never know what's missing.

Motel Cooking

When folks fall from housing to the street they often hit a number of bumps along the way. Many, especially parents of small children, consider themselves lucky if they land a cheap motel room. These no-tell motels require no security deposit and generally charge by the week - requiring less money up front.

One particular mom of seven found herself preparing meals using only a microwave and hot plate. Her are some of those fall-back meals.

Melissa's Quick and Easy Mac and Cheese

- A Package of boxed macaroni and cheese
- Bell peppers
- Bacon bits (real bacon would be such a treat)

Cook macaroni as instructed on the box. Add bacon bits and chopped green pepper. If you have tomato paste, it really makes it special. Mix everything together, add some salt and pepper.

Melissa's Cream Cheese and Chili Dip

This is super quick and easy and very microwave friendly.

- Cream cheese any brand
- Hormel Chili - no beans
- Bag of shredded mild cheddar.

Spread cream cheese on the bottom of microwavable dish. Cover with chile then layer with shredded cheese. Microwave until heated. Serve with chips.

Melissa's Chicken-ish Rice

- One box instant rice
- Can(s) cream of chicken soup

Prepare rice and mix in canned soup. Add some butter if you have it. Add salt, pepper and onion powder.

You can learn more about Melissa and her journey in Diane Nilan and Diana Bowman's excellent book, *The Three Melissas*.

Chapter Four

The Super Bowl

The second most food intensive holiday in America is Super Bowl Sunday. Care to guess what number one is? Yeah, that's right. Thanksgiving. I won't bore you (much) with tales of po' folk Thanksgiving (or Christmas, for that matter) holiday meals. Although I do have one bang-up story about a woman fleeing domestic violence who thought she'd have nothing to eat for Christmas but ending up getting herself a hotdog with money she found on the ground – that story's always a crowd favorite.

See, ordinarily, at the holidays, volunteers rush to help. Swarming end-of-the-year charity dinners, physically serving the same folks they generally forget about – or fear – the rest of the year. Community cupboards or food banks overflow with donated food from mid-November through the end of December.

I was one of those people who made a fuss in late November to collect food and drink for those who have little or none. For five years, as a disc jockey in central Maine, I lived in an A19 M40 Abrams Tank at Camp Keyes Army National Guard base for – wait for it – Tanksgiving! The first year, I lived inside the tank. I had remote radio gear. We ran electrical cords to the tank, and I broadcast live for a full week – 15 hours a day (the other nine hours I tried to sleep) – as National Guard volunteers collected food and cash for those in need.

Funny thing about tons of steel outside, in late autumn, in Maine – it gets damned cold. And by damned, I mean other, much nastier, words. The first year, 2000, the nights were in the teens and the tank was the exact same temperature. It rained during the day and snowed at night. I nearly froze solid. After that first year's glacial experience in a monstrous vehicle that wanted me to be the same temperatures it was, I changed the promotion. Subsequent years, I lived in a tent beside the tank. Still all good fun, but not the same death-defying fight against the elements. Wimping out didn't damage the event's success any either. We still got tons of food and thousands of dollars for those in need.

There are so many stories to tell from our annual Tanksgiving broadcast. We decorated the tank with holiday lights. Had hobo fires and cooked hot dogs over busted-up wooden pallets in a 55-gallon drum. Fire – a great invention! After hours, and between radio breaks, I had free run of the base. I could drop into the NCO club, use the latrine, visit with the guards. That all changed the Tanksgiving after the 9/11 terrorist attacks when the military went on high alert. Post 2001, I had to pass through a guard shack every time I needed a restroom break – and they entirely nixed the rest of my base-wandering ways.

Our biggest paradigm shift came the third year, when we realized that donated food – while vitally important – lacked variety, pizzazz, joie da vivre. That year, one of the station salespeople sold sponsorship of our live radio broadcast to a limousine company. An odd juxtaposition, luxury vehicles and starvation, but we made it work. We asked folks to donate indulgences for dinner. Jars of olives, bottles of sparkling cider, elegant instant desserts. Not only did we get a tankful of regular food: we packed that limo with unnecessary foods that po' folk don't usually get. Capers and Caviar for Christmas and Chanukah!

I'm no anthropologist, so I don't know when our species started to celebrate. Planning events and executing those plans using food, drink, dance and song came somewhere after bipedal walking and before the pyramids. Because our social programing lends itself to sharing the holiday spirit with others, millions of charities have solicited help around those traditional fetes. The knowledge that folks face hardship year-round, and that humans with means feel more compelled to care during holiday seasons, prompted me to invent some imaginary holidays.

When I give talks about homelessness, people invariably ask me what they can do. I always say the same two things: gift cards and imaginary holidays.

Gift cards to fast food joints aren't just great ways to feed others. They also turn the needy into paying customers. And customers can use the restrooms. Talk about a gift!

Imaginary holidays happen when people conjure a new Christmas, Eid Al-Fitr, Passover, Kwanzaa, etc., in their heads. Instead of Thanksgiving being the fourth Thursday in November, a willing participant imagines that it's March 3rd or July 19th – and they volunteer or donate as they would at the more traditional holiday times of the year.

I promise you right now (and I'm sorry that it's true) there will be people burned out of their homes, children without toys, and hungry people every day of every other month of the coming year. There just won't be much competition for you to help them if you pick your own holiday. Most other people will still be focusing on December 25th or the fourth Thursday in November.

Personally, I like to be nice to folks on June 20th. That's my mom's birthday. She's not here for me to be good to, so I do it for someone else. Give it a try – you'll love it.

Where was I? Oh yes, the Super Bowl. Celebrations don't really exist in homeless shelters. Back in the day, when I served as operations manager for that emergency overnight shelter that bedded folks on the floors of churches, I told every new person the same thing. "I bet you if you had your druthers, you wouldn't choose to live with 50 other people." Then pointing toward the common area, I'd add, "And if you did, it wouldn't be this 50!"

Even on the worst day of their lives, I could generally get a smile out of folks with that line.

Sleeping on floors, waiting in line hours for a shower, spending time with folks you don't trust, starting fights, getting robbed, cussed out or insulted: these behaviors don't encourage celebration. Frankly, not much about life in a shelter seems worth celebrating. Which is too bad because celebration is a normal, healthy part of living. Again, I'm no psychologist, but I think it's that lack of normalcy and healthy interaction that makes all other quasi-criminal aspects of homelessness far more likely.

Random, forced cohabitation makes already-cynical residents distrust each other. Street-smart folks don't much trust the employees charged with their care, either. Why would they? The world's dealt shelter-dwellers some rather cruel blows and expecting that to change just because someone's offered to help wastes much-needed hope.

Hope is a tool that the afflicted need for everyday sanity and survival. And hope, by the time someone gets to a shelter, is already in exceedingly short supply.

Were I in their shoes, you wouldn't get a whole pile of optimism out of me, either. It's next-level foolish to give volunteers or minimum-wage employees dominion over other peoples' lives, possessions, firearms and prescriptions. But that's what shelters do.

As a matter of daily routine, our emergency shelter dwellers had to surrender – to total strangers – their weapons or narcotics or both.

Any given night – and every given night – our facility overflowed with abandoned, panicky and angst-ridden folks stressed to their breaking point. If you don't think this sounds like the makings of a perfect Super Bowl party, you need to check that judgment stuff at the door. Because those disaffected, solitary, lonely folks desperately needed someone to suspend the nightly curfew and flick on the game.

Because our shelter relied on church volunteers to open the doors – our rules demanded that all residents report to the resource center and reserve a space on the floor by 8:30 in the evening. The volunteers wanted to get home at a decent hour. In most churches, guests who worked late received special exemption once the shelter verified the worker's schedule.

I'd like you to pause and think about that indignity for a moment. You're poor, you've got no home, and the shelter where you live insists on talking to your boss – or you can just sleep on the street. Many unhoused people fear repercussions at work once their housing status becomes public knowledge. Nice choice – personal privacy or a sleeping mat. Hurry up and pick. You can't have both.

Lots of folks hide their homelessness terrifically well. They masterfully disguise their shame. In fact, I've lost count over the years of all the people we sheltered who, "didn't look homeless." Retired teachers. Little old grandmas. Beautiful, young, pregnant women. Kids who aged out of foster care. Infants. Toddlers. School kids. You get the picture.

Several years ago, a fine young man named Mike walked into our facility. A sweet guy with a sharpish, self-defensive edge, Mike didn't get along with everyone. Some of the shelter staff decided that the handsome, fit, young man thought too much of himself. Some of the other residents got jealous or defensive themselves. A hard worker, Mike took every job that came his way. Often the jobs were menial. He'd finished high school and done a few college classes, but he had no career path and – with a less-than-optimal job climate at the time – Mike took lots of temp jobs. I simply loved the guy.

Yes, Mike had relatives. A single mom off on her own precarious adventure and a remarried dad with a newer, younger set of kids. In my TV days, Kurt Vonnegut spoke at the University of Maine. My press connections got me inside. The *1992 Humanist of the Year* spoke of a disconnected, lonely world, where old disagreements between young adults and their parents could no longer be solved by staying with Uncle Fred. Because Uncle Fred lived a thousand miles away or faced insurmountable struggles of his own, or just didn't exist.

If you read Kurt's speeches, you'll see that he often spoke of guys like Mike. Newly minted adults trying to be themselves in a way that violated the norms their parents demanded they follow. Mike spent more than a few years in need of acceptance but – for circumstances beyond understanding – he couldn't get it at home.

With a story as ordinarily unique as everyone else's, Mike walked through our door. I instantly took to his cynical wit, passion for reading and love of culinary exploration. I never saw that guy without a book. Lots of folks experiencing homelessness seek refuge in libraries. They suck up the WIFI and relatively unconditional acceptance in equal amounts. What often surprises the NIMBY crowd is how many folks experiencing homelessness also read the books!

One of those bibliophiles, Mike read himself to sleep each night. He'd find great passages or beautifully written sentences and he'd text pictures of them to me so I could enjoy them, too. When our paths crossed, we'd talk about food and recipes and, to my dismay – sports! (Well, he talked about sports. I listened).

During one of our conversations in early January, Mike lamented the upcoming Super Bowl game and the shelter policy of sending everyone to their church-floor beds just about the time the second quarter began. "Would there be a way to get televisions set up at the church?" *No, of course not. We had plenty of little kids experiencing homelessness and Super Bowl Sunday is a school night.*

"Let me talk to the boss," I answered. "Perhaps we can have a sign-up for folks who want to stay late."

The next day, I asked the director if we could send some of the "guests" to the church late that night. I volunteered to stay. As did one of our case managers, Stacie Martins (an angel walking the earth if ever there was one). I told the boss that we could use the new Super Bowl privilege as an incentive for guest compliance and orderliness – two things my boss loved, and mass sheltering requires.

A kindhearted soul, the director agreed. Stacie, Mike and I started planning. We posted a sign-up sheet to ascertain which guests wanted to see the Super Bowl. Anyone who wanted to stay at the resource center eating and laughing and watching the game until it ended needed to jot their name on the paper. One of the most curmudgeonly, contrary and short-tempered fellas that ever graced our door signed up first. I went to see him in his corner of the dining area. "Greg, are you sure? You know this means you'll have to do your chores."

He sneered at me, "I will?"

I smiled, "Yeah, you signed up for the Super Bowl party. No chores, no game."

Greg didn't give me the satisfaction of a response – but – he did his chores all month long. Funny what a little respect, dignity and normality will do for a relationship.

In the end, more than twenty of our fifty-or-so shelter-dwellers stayed to watch the game. In addition to the internal sign-up sheet, I solicited the outside world for help. I put a post on Facebook and the homed folks in town bought us hundreds of dollars' worth of food.

Mike made chicken wings and spicy crockpot mac and cheese. Rose (a retired woman with exceptionally bad hips and trouble walking) made taco salad with fresh veggies paid for by strangers. Other folks cooked other things. I can't recall it all. We had snacking foods too. Chips and salsa, iced tea, pickles, hard-boiled eggs and pretzels.

We had no fights. No arguments. No insults. Folks waited on each other. Washed up the dishes. Hooted and hollered for the game.

Mike, Stacie and I had begun turning out fresh hot chicken wings during the pre-game show. Some snacks were shared earlier, so that people who already planned to skip the game could have a few treats. Eventually, moms packed up their children and they and the other disinterested residents headed over to the church.

I worked over the stove, with my back to the television screen. Our partygoers had assembled café-style to watch, yummy food on tables before them. After a few announcements, I heard the *Star-Spangled Banner* begin to play. Stacie tapped my back and I turned around. The entire audience experiencing homelessness stood, with their hands over their hearts. Some even sang along. You could have knocked me down with a feather. A room full of people – living as far as humanly possible from the capitalists' American Dream – stood for the national anthem. I turned back to frying chicken wings, muttering, "These people are too good for this country."

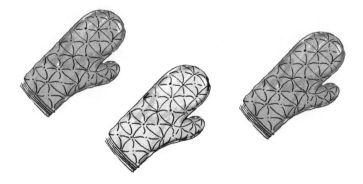

Mike has moved on and is now married to a fantastic woman. They have a wonderful little girl. They've got a comfortable home and a smoker in the backyard. When I contacted him to ask his permission to include him in the book, he told me he doesn't cook that kind of food anymore. "I do a lot of grilled tri-tip now (a cut of beef that's a big part of Santa Monica-style BBQ), smoke a lot of turkey, pulled pork, brisket. Been baking bread, too. Making challah this coming weekend. Also been smoking cheese." Then adding, either because he knew I would want some or at least would want to know more, "I also do a smoked mac and cheese."

After Mike left the shelter and each year after that, Stacie and I continued to do the Super Bowl party at the shelter – even after we'd both stopped working there. Until the pandemic came and life for those experiencing homelessness got universally and exponentially worse.

Mike's Crockpot Spicy Macaroni and Cheese

There are folks who will put Old Bay on anything and everything. It's generally used for seafood – crabs in particular. I'm not a fan, but this was a big hit.

- 1 pound elbow macaroni
- Block Kraft Velveeta Cheese cubed (or the knock off brand)
- Half gallon milk
- Pepper
- Old Bay seasoning (amounts depending on your tastes)

About three hours before you want to serve this – but you can keep it in the crock pot, on low, for lots longer – combine all the ingredients in the pot and cover. Do not pre-cook the pasta.

Stir every half hour.

I have made the same dish with more costly ingredients, substituting brown mustard for the Old Bay. I've used a combination of grated cheddar, gouda, Monterey Jack, Swiss or gruyere. And substituted half the milk with cream. It's *off the charts* good and easy – but about four times as expensive.

Mike's Buffalo Chicken Wings

Meat to money ratio on chicken wings can make this treat cost prohibitive. Luckily for our shelter Super Bowl party, the community chipped in and purchased the ingredients.

- Family pack of chicken wings (you can make fewer, but this is the Super Bowl recipe).
  They are often less expensive if purchasing the whole wing. But then they'll need to be cut apart at the joints.
- Some flour (about a cup – for a family pack)
- Some spices *(Mike didn't remember the exact spices used. Probably garlic, paprika, chili powder, salt, pepper)*
- Cooking oil for frying
- Paper towel or brown paper bag for prep and for draining
- Hot sauce *(brand name like Frank's Red Hot, a generic, or one of the many recipes from the Internet)*
- Blue cheese dressing
- Celery and carrot sticks

Wash the chicken wings and place on a paper towel. In a bowl or plastic bag mix flour and dry spices. Coat the chicken wings in spiced flour. If using a plastic bag, this is really quite easy. Put wings in the bag and shake until all the wings are coated. Heat oil on medium high on the stove. When oil is 375 degrees Fahrenheit (or when a water droplet pops if you drop it into the oil) – place chicken wings in and cook until brown. Don't overcrowd the oil. Fry in batches and allow oil to return to 375 degrees between batches. *(If you're a seasoned cook you likely already know this… but for the sake of those who aren't…* **Be very careful with hot oil. Neglected oil can start a very hazardous fire. Never attempt to put a hot oil fire out with water. Always cover to smother the flame).**

Drain on brown paper, then put in clean, empty bowl and pour hot sauce on top. Shake until coated. Serve wings with celery and carrot sticks and blue cheese dressing.

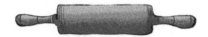

Mike's life is completely different today. He's got a great job. He belongs to the union where he works – which anecdotally is the single biggest indicator that you'll never be homeless. *Although one of the old men at the Super Bowl party proved the exception to the rule. He'd worked for Bethlehem Steel and when they went belly-up, the laws passed during the Reagan administration allowed the company to stiff the workers on their retirement. Our elderly veteran experiencing homelessness lived on ten percent of his pension. His monthly check should have been $2780. Instead, he received a meager $278 per month.*

Mike sent along a recipe from his new life to share with you here. He said it's a very affordable cut of meat and makes a delicious anchor to any meal. You'll need a meat thermometer to cook the way Mike does now.

Mike's Pork Shoulder Recipe

- 1 pork shoulder
- 4 heads of garlic
- 4 tablespoons oregano
- 2 tablespoons black pepper
- 4 tablespoons extra virgin olive oil
- 4 tablespoons adobo *(The Spice House has a lovely variety)*

- 2 packets of sazon (Loisa brand is nice)
- 1 cup sour orange juice (usually found, bottled, in the international section of the grocery store)

"Mix wet and dry ingredients and coat the shoulder. Refrigerate several hours or overnight. Place in a Dutch oven or other covered pot and roast at 350 until the internal temperature hits 180. Turn heat up to 450 and roast until the internal temp is 203. *All of the above spice mixtures recommended can be made from scratch fairly easily if you have an ample spice rack.*"

Also, if you're looking for a great spice company to buy everything from, I can't recommend Penzeys enough.

Chapter Five

Geralyn

Geralyn thought the Bangor, Maine police loved her. She appreciated that they dropped by the overnight lot where she parked and slept and ate and read and relieved herself and… well, you get the picture.

She thought they liked her and – knowing Geralyn – they probably did. But their real reason for morning visits was to make sure that any frozen, dead bodies were removed from public places at the department's earliest possible convenience. In a region where January's overnight temperatures average in the single digits Fahrenheit, the authorities knew it was best to check all the outdoor sleepers each morning – first thing.

Geralyn was lovable. Heck, the first 20 plus years I knew her we managed to be absolutely crazy about each other via email, my radio program and the occasional phone call. Someone might have predicted we'd be besties – she with her rapier wit and me with my soft spot for the needy and fervent passion for people who make me laugh.

The Bangor police, on the other hand, had a far more checkered past with those experiencing homelessness. That's not unique for law enforcement organizations. They're often instructed by elected officials to treat homelessness as a crime. Although, sometimes, the cops – like other folks in life – just don't like the folks who live on the edge.

One time, the Bangor police ticked me off so bad – with their insensitivity and boorish arrogance toward the down and out – that I organized a picket of the police station and drove nearly 600 miles – all the way from Carlisle, Pennsylvania – to lead it. If you don't already know the mid-Atlantic commonwealths from the New England states, buy a map. That's a long ride around some rather busy cities and the traffic is brutal.

I'm not picking on cops. And I'm not talking *they used to be uneven-handed with the poor.* I'm talking **still**. A couple of years ago the authorities in Bangor shoved some outside sleepers out of the public eye so vehemently that the men hid in an abandoned building to escape their harassment. Later that same evening the building caught fire and the men died. Every last one of them!

That's just one example. Similar tragedies happen across the nation. And will happen even more often now that the Supreme Court of the United States ruled that municipalities could make homelessness illegal. (You know the drill. See the bibliography for info on Grants Pass v. Johnson).

Let's face it – especially with SCOTUS bestowing carte blanche on cruelty – our police departments will improperly respond to people in crisis. And it won't stop until we start understanding the nature of homelessness and the purpose of law enforcement as they have evolved in the United States. When the police respond to anything, any call at all, they bring with them lethal force. It's their training, and, therefore, their go-to solution. And it's literally deadly. America needs a peace-keeping branch of government that responds in person to situations of dire need with blankets, not bullets. Patience, not patrol cars. And tenderness, not tasers. We aren't there yet. In fact, we're working backwards. Ruthless cops aren't the only ones to blame for our lousy response to human crisis. They get their marching orders from civilians who disregard and disrespect the needs of the unhoused. Consequently, the cops aren't equipped to help.

Allow me to digress a bit more and explain the 2024 SCOTUS ruling. Seems a little town in Oregon passed an ordinance that anyone with visible intention of sleeping outside – a pillow, blanket, cardboard – (I'm sure Geralyn had all of these), would be ticketed and fined. After a certain number of unpaid fines, they'd be banished from the town limits. If they did not get out – and stay out – they'd face charges, get locked up, and incur more debt.

Just what a person in homelessness needs! A criminal record, debt and to lose all their belongings when the cops haul them out of their unstable living situation.

This rather pure form of cruelty was challenged in court by a collection of people living rough in the community. Gloria Johnson was the lead name on the class-action lawsuit. After the plaintiffs won in the 9th circuit court of appeals, Grants Pass ponied up the money to ask the Supreme Court for relief.

The 9th circuit judges had ruled that punishing people for something they had no choice about, was wrong. (Using the example – if you broke into a store to escape a hurricane, it's not illegal). So, yeah, Grants Pass, unable to learn their lesson from the 9th circuit, appealed it to the highest court in the land.

A lot rode on that decision. The state of Florida and many other smaller jurisdictions were hoping to get away with criminalizing homelessness if the SCOTUS decided this case wrongly. The shocker came, not when SCOTUS – now peppered with cruel, ignorant, out-of-touch justices supported the selfishness of Grants Pass. The head rocking I'm doing now is that "liberal" California has proven to be as heartless as any other U.S. jurisdiction. State and local authorities have put more than 2000 homeless camps on the chopping block because – well – now they can. That ruling, tragically flawed as it is, poses cataclysmic consequences for the Geralyns of the world.

Let's learn more about Geralyn.

Geralyn worked the comedy circuit in New York. Ate pizza with George Carlin. Sold a bit to Robin Williams. "One he used on Johnny Carson when Johnny was still host," she'd confide proudly, if you'd take the time to listen. She did her own stand-up routines, too. But mostly she hung around the clubs, selling gags and one-liners to other comedians.

She liked them all, but Williams the most, "He and I used humor for the same thing – protection!"

Geralyn often spoke about herself or family members when she wrote, "I'm studying to be agoraphobic. The homework's a cinch, but graduation will be a bitch."

Often her jokes seemed to be about random people, but they were inspired by the uncomfortable relationships in her own life. When we were alone, she explained it this way, "My mother never understood me, but she never tried."

In public, to elicit the humor that fed her soul, her barbs took on a generic tone. "She had an inferiority complex so good, she actually made herself inferior."

Like Williams, humor could only protect her so far. She fell victim to her mental illness and died way too early after living a decade or more on the street.

For a while after her time living in her car, and before her final eviction, Geralyn had some good years. Well-educated and a born performer, Geralyn's life stabilized when, after years of red tape, the U.S. federal government approved her disability. Motivated by her feelings of intense gratitude, Geralyn reached out to others – she spoke regularly about the horrors of poverty and homelessness.

When Geralyn spoke to the housed, she used words. When she spoke to the unhoused, she used food.

Geralyn gave back to others by cooking for the shelter that rescued her from her car. She showed compassion by listening to others experiencing homelessness and, whenever possible, she'd cook the foods she liked best. Figuring if she liked it, most of them would, too.

"It wasn't easy. You had to depend on the food that got donated. I'd prepare dinner twice a week. I'd go in the day before and take some sort of protein out of the walk-in freezer and give it time to thaw. The next day I'd pull together something tasty." Geralyn smiled as she spoke about cooking for neighbors in need.

"When you donate to a soup kitchen, don't forget spices. Food can get awfully bland without it. I knew some folks who liked food that way, so if I had spices, I'd prepare about half the way I would have eaten it and the other half as plain as possible." Geralyn, who hailed from the deep south, added, "Louisianans like food with some kick."

Most of Geralyn's recipes land in the next chapter – the one about soup kitchens. But this one, her personal favorite, is a gift from her to you. No shelter in Bangor, Maine, (or most other places, I'll wager) ever got catfish on a scale that made this recipe possible.

Before the comedienne-turned-cook got a home of her own, she'd doubled up with a few other folks in need. When she had the disposable income, she'd make this catfish treat for them. When I asked her for recipes for this book, she wanted me to make sure you – someone learning about her for the first time – got this one!

One last thing about G. I'd hoped to dedicate this book to her. I told her so, on her deathbed. She told me, "No!" She didn't ask me not to do it, mind you. She ordered me. "Don't dedicate it to me. Dedicate it to hungry people." So I did.

Beer & Corn Meal Batter Fried Catfish

(Recipe copied directly from Geralyn's email, commentary and all)

Honestly, I don't think I've made this since I made it for "the boys" when I was in transitional housing. I ended up having to read several other fried catfish recipes and cobbling this together, using what sounded right. Since I was raised Cajun, we mix stuff together until we can say "That looks right" and take it from there. If you try making this, let me know if it works!

- 1-1.5 pounds catfish or other fish
  (would not recommend with haddock)
- 1/2 cup all-purpose flour
- 1/2 cup corn meal
- 1 tablespoon garlic powder
- 1 teaspoon baking powder
- 1 teaspoon paprika
- 2 tablespoons Cajun seasoning
- 1 egg
- 3/4 cup beer (room-temperature and flat)
  vegetable oil for frying
  For the fish:
- 1/2 teaspoon salt (or Cajun seasoning)
- 1/3 cup buttermilk or milk

Instructions

CATFISH:

- Mix together the 1/2 tsp salt (or Cajun seasoning) and buttermilk or milk. Soak fillets in this mixture while preparing the batter.
- In a medium bowl, mix together flour, cornmeal, baking powder, and all your spices. Add your beer and egg and mix well, until everything is incorporated. Refrigerate for at least 30 minutes to help everything set.

- When ready to cook, pour vegetable oil in a fryer or deep skillet to a depth of at least 3 inches, and heat to 375°.
- Allow fillets to drip dry then flip-flop them on a paper towel to insure they are not wet. Dip fillets in batter, lifting with tongs and letting excess batter drip off.
- When the oil is hot, draining excess batter, place battered catfish in oil, several pieces at a time using tongs (do not overcrowd fillets).
- Fry until browned, about 3-4 minutes.
- Remove to paper towels to drain excess oil and repeat with remaining fish.
- To keep warm while you fry the rest of the fish, place on a baking sheet and keep in a low, warmed oven (150°-200°)

Beer Batter Hushpuppies

Down south, I think it's a law that you must serve hush puppies with fried catfish. I'm not sure. Remember, as noted below, you can fry the hush puppies in the same oil you did the fish. I do... you're going to eat them together, after all!

- Total: 20 min
- Prep: 5 min
- Cook: 15 min
- Yield: 15 hushpuppies

- About 4 cups canola oil, for frying
- 2 cups white or yellow cornmeal
- 2 teaspoons baking powder
- Pinch of cayenne pepper (I, of course, use Cajun seasoning, and more than a pinch)
- 1 cup beer, (flat and room-temp, plus more, if needed)
- 2 large eggs
- 1 onion, very finely chopped
- 1/2 C parsley (if desired), minced

Directions

- In a large cast-iron Dutch oven, heat the oil over high heat until it reaches 375 degrees F on a deep-fry thermometer. (You can fry the hush puppies in the same oil you did the fish. I do... you're going to eat them together, after all!)
- To make the batter, in a large bowl whisk together the

cornmeal, baking powder, and seasonings. In a second bowl or large liquid measuring cup, combine the beer, eggs and onions. Add the seasonings and whisk until smooth. Stir the wet ingredients into the dry ingredients, using as few strokes as possible. (The mixture should resemble wet sand; add more beer, if needed.)

- Line a plate with paper towels and set by the cooktop. To fry the hushpuppies, scoop up the batter using a medium ice cream scoop or a soup ladle (half full) and drop it into the hot oil without crowding.
- Fry, stirring occasionally with a slotted spoon, until golden brown, 3 to 5 minutes. Remove with a slotted spoon to the prepared plate. Adjust the heat to maintain the proper temperature and repeat with the remaining batter. Serve immediately.

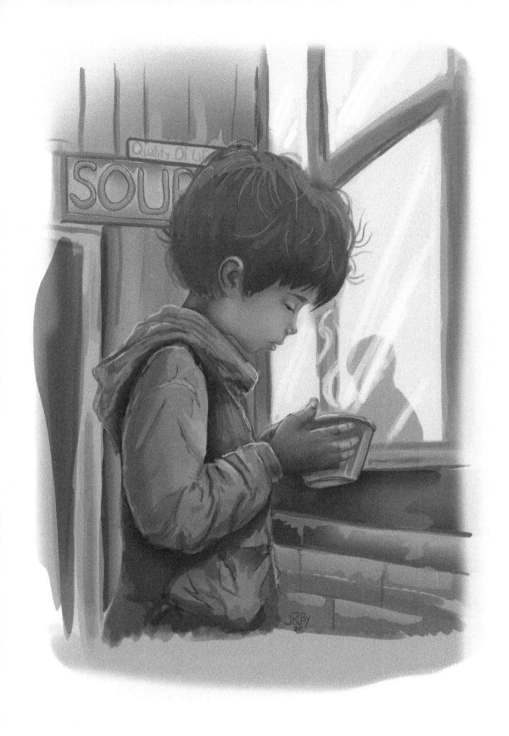

Interventions

Chapter Six

Eating Crow

The United States – the wealthiest nation on earth – has hundreds of thousands of soup kitchens. While exact figures aren't available, Encyclopedia dot com names Second Harvest as the largest private feeding network in the nation, supplying more than 94,000 soup kitchens and food pantries.

Many branches of the federal government supply funding for communal mass feeding. Even the Department of Housing and Urban Development has, over the years, subsidized public feeding programs if the would-be recipients could prove they were experiencing homelessness. The inability to prove a negative – that one doesn't have a home, according to HUD's narrow definition – leaves an awful lot of people without support.

In addition to non-secular organizations as well as state and federal agencies, nearly half of all U.S. faith-based entities have supplemental feeding programs. In the U.S., people's tummies are hurting and nearly every church, mosque, synagogue, school department, and local municipality knows it. Yet effective, long-term solutions to the problem of food insecurity meet fierce pushback – think housing and Grants Pass.

With hundreds of thousands of diverse entities stepping up to feed the community, it's a wonder the problem persists. But the scope is that enormous. Additionally, hunger and malnutrition continue to plague the nation because, while many work diligently to feed their neighbors, others prefer to move them out of sight and push them further out of town – hiding the problem entirely, when possible.

In 2011, I ventured into Gainesville, Florida with my activist co-conspirator, Diane Nilan. Diane and I have traveled together for nearly a decade and a half. During our sojourns, we gather data and school interested parties on the reality that faces people in homelessness and poverty across the wealthiest nation on earth. We included our trip to gator country when we ventured into the U.S. southeast on a trip we dubbed *The Southern Discomfort Tour.*

Every now and then we find areas and agencies doing a better job than anywhere else. More often than we'd care to recall, we find organizations and municipalities failing miserably and sloppily hiding their cruelty.

When Diane and I suspect malice, we seldom announce our arrival. Consequently, Gainesville didn't know we were coming. If they had, they likely wouldn't have extended a warm welcome. After all, they're merciless to their own neighbors who suffer in silence and we have a habit of running our mouths.

One January day we showed up around noon at the St. Francis House Soup Kitchen. We were greeted by ten or so fresh, young faces at the food service line. Members of the University of Florida's Circle K club – a division of Kiwanis International – stood before pans full of food, eager to feed the needy. Other than these volunteers, the room was empty. Poised with ladles in hand, they asked us to sign a sheet with numbered spaces so they could feed us.

There we stood, at lunch time, at a soup kitchen in a city of more than 120,000 people and there wasn't a single person eating.

We asked for the kitchen manager. Michael Robles walked over and introduced himself. I said, "We hear there's a limit on how many people you can feed here at St. Francis." Robles confirmed the rumor.

In fact, Robles told us, no matter how much food he had, no matter how many nice kids volunteered to help, no matter how many hours he was willing to stay open, and no matter how many hungry people came to the door, the soup kitchen was not to feed more than 130 people.

About a year and a half earlier, the Gainesville city commissioners decided to enforce a decades-old regulation that restricted St. Francis House. The ordinance forbade the soup kitchen to allow more than 130 individuals to eat there. Robles explained that neither he nor the rest of the shelter staff had actually seen the "on the books" regulation. He said that while enforced as though it were in print somewhere, the regulation appeared to be "off the books" and no city leader has ever produced proof of its existence.

Still, city commissioners reminded Robles that if he fed 131 people, his kitchen would be shut down. Everyone would go hungry, instead of just the handful that get rejected when the feeding quota is met. Secondarily, Robles knew that if the commissioners made good on their threat, he – a single dad – would need to look for work.

St. Francis House Soup Kitchen is just part of the overall St. Francis House outreach – making the feeding limit even more perplexing. As confused as we were, Robles pointed out that the feeding limit was too small, even for the participants in their other programs. He explained, "Because the shelter half of this building serves 280 people a day with showers, mailboxes, phones, messages and hygiene products, we could probably feed 400," including random town folk.

Robles estimates a fair and adequate number would be even higher because individuals and families don't have to be homeless to be hungry. "On one of my toughest days, a mom came in with her two kids and we had already fed 128 people. I told her that she put us over the top. She said, 'Well, just feed my kids and I won't eat.' And that's what we had to do. We piled those two trays really high, though." Robles smiled, "If the kids couldn't finish what they had, well I guess they took it home."

Robles gave us a tour of his soup kitchen facility. We stood in an overflowing food storage room. I asked why the city commissioners would so hardheartedly enforce such a ridiculous rule when there were plenty of hungry people and the soup kitchen had plenty of food.

Robles speculated, "It's about zoning." Once at the outskirts of the city, St. Francis House is now in the heart of downtown Gainesville – an anchor building surrounded by rundown workforce housing in an area only recently converted from septic systems to a public sewer.

Robles continued, "Developers want this area. Look across the street. They've built a dog park! They care more for their dog recreation facilities than they do for the people."

It doesn't take a whole lot of deductive reasoning to figure out that hunger – the most curable plague in the U.S. – persists by design. It's the same for homelessness. Hunger and homelessness keep the barely fed and barely housed from complaining.

If someone can barely pay the rent, they keep quiet because… well… at least they can pay the rent. If someone can barely feed their family, they keep quiet because… well… at least they can feed their family. The *don't make waves – things could get worse* philosophy suits the needs of power retailers and fast-food giants. Desperation and a fear of increasing hardship keeps folks working for low wages with few arguments. At least until recently.

Sometimes things get bad enough, and the workers band together, organize and succeed. Amazon and Starbucks workers in 2022 started feeling more powerful and things for them have begun changing. United Auto Workers (UAW) accomplishments in the south, where 30% of U.S. automotive workers are employed, have engendered hope that labor unions may have more success organizing. Wage increases associated with the pandemic shook things up as well – but we'll get to that later. The pandemic gets a whole chapter of its own.

The end of the story is – people who pay too much for rent, healthcare and other necessities can't afford to feed themselves. Until disability benefits, social security payments, wages and gig jobs start producing a living wage, soup kitchens and food pantries will endure.

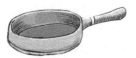

My friend G, after being rescued from homelessness by the Greater Bangor Area Homeless Shelter, started volunteering to feed the folks in the adjacent soup kitchen twice a week. Although I hadn't met her at the time, I volunteered at the exact same place – cooking for forty or so hungry people, one night a month. I generally took a recipe I made at home for my family and made ten times the amount. My mom paid for the food. I just cooked it.

G didn't have a benefactor to pay for the food she prepared at the shelter. She would scrounge around in the donations closets and fridges and create meals based on what she found in stock. Here are some of the tips that G said helped her when cooking for large numbers. I'll put her exact words in italics.

Stuff I learned (and realized) while cooking for the Shelter

It's important to visit the shelter pantry the day before. Some proteins will have to be set out to defrost (chicken, ham, etc.) and to plan. You need an idea of what you've got to work with the next day. I've found that it's also good to gather all the stuff you've picked out, box it together and mark it clearly with the date and which meal it's going to be used for, as well as your name. This saves you from having to scramble the next day when someone's taken off with your ham or other necessary ingredient.

If using a mixture of fresh, canned and frozen veggies for a dish, remember you'll have to cook the fresh veggies first, on their own, as they take a little longer to cook and you'll need a little extra time to prep them.

It's probably best to avoid a lot of garlic, onions, and peppers (any color) as some people's digestive systems can be sensitive. For instance, in my personal cooking, I go by the adage There's no such thing as too much garlic! But, in cooking for others, I rein that in. I use just enough for a little garlic flavor, but not any more than that. Same for onions and peppers.

Celery adds bulk, good fiber and cooks down to thicken gravies and sauces. Added parsley is always nice, if you have it. It also adds dash of color and cooks down quickly.

Go easy on the spices. Offer hot sauce and salt and pepper on the tables (when possible) and never get your nose bent out of shape when people use ketchup or ask for other condiments. Different strokes for different folks!

It's a shame, but a lot of "group friendly" recipes are heavy on carbohydrates. Again, not good for some health issues, but very, very filling, and, of course, a classic comfort food. That's why potato-based recipes and anything over pasta or rice (or other grains) is handy when cooking for a group. When faced with cooking something like that, I tend to try to go overboard on the meat (when possible) and veggies, to counterbalance. For instance, a ham and scalloped potato casserole works just fine when you can double up on the meat and add frozen peas to give folks a little more nutrition.

I was raised Cajun and taught the "Trinity" method of cooking. Every recipe needs onion, bell pepper and celery. Through the years,

I dropped the bell pepper and added parsley and/or garlic. These four items have become the basis for most of my large group recipes.

I learned that it's always good to have a big pot of just veggies. A mix of broccoli, cauliflower, carrots, or just run-of-the-mill mixed veggies on the side is a great mass feeding supplement.

Besides, there ARE vegan homeless. Additionally, I personally just craved vegetables when eating off 'the kindness of strangers'.

Use your imagination. A can of beets in the fridge makes a good dessert when you're craving something sweet.

One of G's favorite Group-Friendly
'Reverse-Engineered Recipes'
Chicken Stew

Eight servings – multiply accordingly for larger crowds

- 4 chicken breasts, roasted & chopped
- 2 C mushrooms
- 4 C mixed veg (If using a mixture of fresh, canned and frozen veggies, remember to cook the fresh veggies first, on their own)
- 1 can condensed cream of mushroom soup
- 1 can condensed cream of chicken soup (cream of celery works, too – you don't even taste the celery, and you get the creamy effect)
- 8 boiling onions or 1 onion, chopped coarsely
- 4 cloves garlic, minced
- ½ bunch of parsley, chopped fine
- ½ head of celery, chopped fine
- Salt and pepper to taste

Combine all the ingredients in a large pot and bring to a boil. Reduce the heat and cook for an hour (if you have the time) to combine flavors. Sautéing vegetables in oil or butter beforehand can add flavor and reduce simmering time.

This can also be stretched by adding pasta or serving over rice. You can also mix up some biscuit mix and milk and cook up some dumplings in this for variety but be prepared for people asking for seconds and thirds on the dumplings – they are classic comfort food.

G's Hamburger Stew

Eight servings – multiply accordingly for larger crowds

- 2 lbs. ground hamburger (can also use stew meat or roast(s), cooked & chopped up)
- 2 8 oz. containers beef broth
- 2 C mushrooms
- 2 C mixed vegetables
- 1 can condensed cream of mushroom soup
- 8 boiling onions quartered or 1 onion, chopped coarsely
- 4 cloves garlic, minced
- ½ clump of parsley, chopped fine
- ½ head of celery, chopped fine
- Salt and pepper to taste

(can also be stretched by adding pasta or serving over rice)

Cook onions, garlic, celery along with the beef. Use a smidgen of oil if the beef is lean. Add mushrooms and mixed veggies, then the cream of mushroom soup and broth. Simmer until thick.

'Semi Cajun' Red Beans & Rice

(for every 4 servings)

I call it semi-Cajun because you can rarely get the 'right' sausage up here in Maine. There was a little squawking about the beans not being 'sweet' (which would knock the 'Cajun' right out of the recipe name), but everyone cleaned their plates, and a LOT of folks came back for seconds.

- 1 lb. dried red beans (or black beans or mix 'em) (follow instructions & soak overnight) - (when using canned beans, count on 2 cans per person, so 8 cans here sub for 1 lb. dried beans)
- 2 lbs. smoked sausage (preferably Cajun, but that's hard to find and pricey up in Maine, so any kind of smoked sausage) Substitute: chopped cooked ham, any kind of pork (roast, chops, even country ribs), cooked low & slow, then shredded.
- 1 purple onion, chopped small
- 2 cloves garlic, minced
- 2 peppers (green, red, yellow, whatever), chopped small
- 1 head of celery, chopped fine (gives bulk & fiber)
- 1/2 bunch of parsley, cut fine

- 2 8 oz. containers beef broth (or veggie broth, even chicken)
- 2 cans chopped tomatoes (or fresh)
- Salt and pepper to taste

Instructions

- After beans have been soaked (if necessary), brown the onion, garlic, peppers, celery and parsley (and tomatoes, if using fresh) in butter or olive oil until translucent and/or wilted, then add cooked meat – sauté just long enough to mix thoroughly.
- Add beans and liquid, then stir regularly on a low simmer until beans are tender.
- Make a big pot of rice (or several smaller pots of rice) while beans are simmering.

Serve beans over rice.

Tuna Casserole

- 4 servings
- 4 cans of tuna (drain all, especially if they're the 'in oil' variety)
- 2 lbs. pasta (any variety - you can use different varieties together, just keep in mind different types may require different cooking times)
- 1 can condensed cream of mushroom soup
- 1 can condensed cream of celery soup
- 3 C vegetables (fresh, canned, frozen, just keep in mind fresh takes a little longer to cook, so you can start them separately first) ... good choices: peas, corn, carrots, green beans, lima beans
- 1 head of celery, chopped fine
- ½ purple onion, chopped fine
- 2 cloves garlic, minced
- ½ bunch of parsley, minced
- 2 C diced cheese (or shredded), whatever you can get your hands on.

Bread crumbs, cracker crumbs or smashed croutons—whichever you have

Cook the fresh veggies together first, while the pasta is boiling (or cook them together – like carrots, etc.).

After the pasta is done, drain and return to pot. Add rest of the veggies, the condensed soup and either a water-milk (1 to 1) mixture or reconstituted coffee creamer (yeah, really) to make it 'saucy'

After that has simmered together a little and been mixed thoroughly, spoon into baking pans.

Top with bread or cracker crumbs (or even smashed croutons) and cheese and slip into the oven (350 degrees) just until the cheese gets melty and the bread crumbs brown just a little.

Turkey Pot Pie

A friend of mine (after I was past being homeless) bought 3 turkeys around the holidays one year and we worked together to make turkey pot pies. She was in charge of the pastry part, so I don't really have a recipe for that, but it was basically my chicken stew recipe, and we cooked the turkeys beforehand and chopped the meat all up. We added the turkey 'juices' along with cream of celery and cream of mushroom soup (to retain the turkey flavor. We ended up making FOUR big pans and took it to the shelter (we'd let them know we were coming beforehand). It was a big hit and we ended up running a little short!

Bonus recipe – I'm going to leave my turkey pie recipe here, too – in case you don't have one. There's nothing too dramatically different about it than anyone else's I'm sure – except that I try to incorporate all the leftovers. I don't believe I've ever made a turkey pie without roasting a turkey first. But, like Geralyn indicated above: if you're cooking for 40 people you won't be using leftovers, you'll be starting from scratch.

- Leftover Turkey meat, cut bite-sized
- Leftover mashed potatoes
- Leftover stuffing
- Leftover peas
- Leftover gravy
- 1 onion, chopped
- 4 stalks celery, chopped
- 4 tablespoons butter
- Salt pepper
- 1 pie crust

Archie the Pie Guy has a great crust recipe. His is the last section in the book. My mom had a very simple pie recipe. Also, Pillsbury pre-made crusts in the grocery store's refrigerated section are delish and functional. And, yes, I've tried the generic versions of the pre-made

– they don't meet my standards, but Pillsbury does. My kids give me a hard time when I use them, but for a pie made of leftovers, using them makes life so simple.

Line the bottom of a pie plate with the one crust. You may also use a casserole dish. Pre-heat the oven to 350. Melt butter in a pan and sauté celery and onions. If you don't have much gravy left, you might want to add flour to the sautéed celery and onions, then add water and get a gravy going. By all means, add leftover drippings and gravy, if you have them, for improved flavor.

Put bite-sized turkey and leftover veggies – especially peas – in the pie shell. Pour your homemade gravy all over it. Then use leftover mashed potato and stuffing to make the top shell. I just cover the top of the pie with tablespoon amounts of each, alternating like a checkerboard. Bake about 40 minutes to an hour or until heated through.

Bonus recipe – *My mom made sausage stuffing. I have tried making other kinds. But, seriously, what's the point? There's nothing better than sausage stuffing. She used it to stuff anything. Stuffed fresh pork shoulder, stuffed chicken, stuffed turkey – you name it. See the stuffing recipe below.*

If it's possible to get freshly made sausage, do so. If you're in Maine, use Mailhot's Best. And after doing a quick web search I see that this Lewiston, Maine-made treat is available in select locations around the country. It's worth a try to find it near you.

If you want to be risqué you may use spicy Italian sausage. There is literally no sausage I've ever tried that isn't perfect for this.

Genevieve's Irish Sausage Stuffing

- 1 lb. pork sausage of your choosing
- 1 or 2 large onions
- 6 long stalks (or more) celery
- ¼ lb. of butter
- Pepper
- 4 cups bread cut into cubes or one bag stuffing mix

Melt butter in large skillet and sauté chopped onions and celery. Add pepper while cooking. When fully cooked, move to large bowl and use same pan to brown the sausage. Add to bowl with vegetables. Toast the cubed bread in the over at 300 degrees for five minutes or use bag of stuffing mix. Add bread to bowl and stir. Spoon mixture into whatever you're stuffing. You can also pound chicken breasts flat. Place a spoonful of stuffing in the center and roll. Secure with toothpicks and bake at 350 for 30 minutes.

Chapter Seven
After School

The United States Department of Agriculture (USDA) has funding and supports for after- school feeding programs. Individual school departments as well as public or private after-school programs that cater to the needs of youth from economically disadvantaged families may access funding and resources. Some school departments, Boys and Girls Clubs, YMCA or YWCA programs – and others – do a bang-up job getting extra calories into kids who would otherwise go hungry.

Some do not.

Feeding programs that rely on freshly cooked food are labor-intensive and require a firm commitment from the organization providing meals. Many of the organizations tasked with caring for poor kids before and after school just don't have the financial wherewithal to add staff or expensive fresh foodstuffs which would increase their expenses.

One organization – the Kids' Kitchen at The Boys and Girls Club in Waterville, Maine (officially called Boys & Girls Clubs and YMCA of Greater Waterville at the Alfond Youth & Community Center) – under the leadership of Eva Grover did commit itself to providing delicious fresh food and a whole lot more.

Here's how it worked: Waterville, Maine is a small town on the Kennebec River in the central part of the state. About 16,000 people live there and by Maine standards they are young. You see, Maine's got the oldest population in the country and Waterville's per capita elderly population is lower than the state average. These young people have young people, and in the early 2000s, about 20% of those kids lived below the poverty level. One thing about poor kids — especially the children of the working poor — is that they are usually pretty hungry by the end of the day.

Poverty is directly related to food insecurity. And according to the Urban Institute's paper on *Feeding America, Feeding Low-Income Children*, food insecurity among children is responsible for "health problems, education problems, and workforce and job readiness problems."

Children who go home to houses with little or no food in the cupboard often have a working parent who is absent part of the time, as well. In 2010, a full 36 percent of the families Feeding America served had at least one working family member. That's a pretty old statistic, and without more recent public numbers we'll just have to do a little math. Because of the great recession of 2009, the Bureau of Labor Statistics stated that the unemployment rate in December of 2010 was 9.4 percent. Lots of those 2010 families were out of work. If we use today's labor stats (2024) with their 4.2 percent unemployment – chances are that about 80 percent of families have at least one working family member now.

The children in Waterville, Eva Grover's stomping ground, were no more immune to the negative effects of poverty, food insecurity and work-related absentee parenting than kids in other parts of the country might be. But they did have a remedy that other communities did not. They had the Kids' Kitchen. Every child who went to the youth center after school was given a hearty, healthy meal – often the last one many children ate each day.

Quite a few children got their first meal there, too. Eva and her staff prepared breakfasts as well.

In 2002, while working as a radio broadcaster in the Central Maine – Waterville area, I was invited to dine at the Kids' Kitchen and meet the founder. I drove in a blinding blizzard to broadcast my morning show. Walking in from the storm, a feisty retired nurse greeted me. Eva had, several years earlier, decided to feed every hungry kid she met while volunteering at the Waterville Boy and Girls Club (which it was called when she started).

I did a regular bit on my show about great places to eat breakfast. I generally broadcast live from the diners and restaurants that our show's fans recommended. After months of airing the weekly segment, I got the phone call telling me about a tiny older woman (under five feet tall) who made a giant difference in the lives of the children around her. I promised the caller that I would check out breakfast at the Kids' Kitchen the following Friday.

I expected a relatively humdrum broadcast that morning because blizzards tend to slow things down at most businesses. Because the blizzard weather made driving treacherous, if I'd broadcast from a diner, I might have been the only customer there. The exact opposite was the case at the Alfond Youth Center. The center housed a combined local YMCA after/before school program along with the Boys and Girls Club's programs. When school got cancelled – as it had been that day – working parents still had to work. Consequently, the Kids' Kitchen overflowed with children long before I arrived.

Walking beside a child the staff had sent to escort me, I followed my nose. Sniffing bacon and sausage, I went down a long hallway that led to an eight-burner stove where Eva stood, feverishly preparing meals for about sixty children. Another five older women walked back and forth through the dining room serving the children their breakfast.

Feeling puckish, I sat at a table alongside several "other" hungry kids. I waited patiently for my turn to speak with the organization's founder. While there, I interviewed a number of the children and marveled at the quiet, orderly way in which the operation around me functioned.

One of the grandmotherly waitresses asked a little boy seated next to me what he wanted for breakfast. The tyke, about six-years-old, responded, "Scrambled eggs." The woman didn't budge. An older, more experienced patron – a girl about twelve years of age – leaned down to whisper in the boy's ear, "You have to say, 'please,' or they won't move." The young fella corrected himself, "Scrambled eggs, please." And off his waitress trotted to fulfill his request.

After the children finished eating and left for their various activities, Eva caught a minute to sit down. She explained that her goal wasn't just to feed the children a meal that one might expect to get at home. She also intended to mirror all the lessons they would have learned at home, during that mealtime. Eva believed that proper etiquette and manners were as important (maybe even more so) to kids from economically disadvantaged families as they were to any other child.

I asked Eva how she got involved with the operation in the first place. Holding my broadcast mic in front of her – live on the radio, she explained, "It started when I volunteered at the Boys and Girls Club. I was a retired nurse and I got bored sitting at home." Eva explained that she'd wait out front of the building for the children to get off the bus and welcome them into the afterschool program and, "some of the little ones said that they were hungry."

Grover went to the store and bought the fixings for peanut butter and jelly sandwiches. She fed the children who were there that first day and planned to do the same the next day. "But I couldn't." Eva stared wide-eyed as she explained that she didn't have enough food. "The next day there were twice as many kids waiting for me." Word had gotten out that this kind old lady at the youth center would feed the children. "I knew then that an awful lot of the children in the community were hungry."

Within a few years, and after hundreds of thousands of dollars donated by Maine philanthropists Harold and Bibby Alfond, what started as a personal gift of sandwich makings for a dozen hungry kids had grown to a youth feeding program making more than 40,000 meals each year. (And now – twelve years after her death – Eva's program feeds nearly 100,000 meals each year).

In 2002, Eva Grover was inducted into the Alfond Youth Center Hall of Fame. Shortly thereafter, well into her seventies, Eva retired from her second and best-loved profession, cooking for the poorest kids in her community.

But again, she couldn't sit still. Shifting her attention to the American Red Cross, Eva traveled the nation helping at hurricanes and other disasters. She deployed to Louisiana in the wake of Hurricane Katrina.

To this day, one of my favorite Eva stories involved none other than former Secretary of State, Colin Powell. At a time when the four-star general considered a career in politics, he made a goodwill trip to visit various parts of Maine. Powell added to his itinerary a not-so-politically-connected place – the Alfond Youth Center.

Powell walked into Eva's kitchen and asked her if he might have, "One of her famous peanut butter and jelly sandwiches." She offered to prepare him one with all the care and love she'd put in every child's meal. He said, "Not necessary." Then the general sat at a table where some of the children were already eating and helped himself to a sandwich from the plate she'd piled high for the children who didn't like whatever hot meal she'd prepared that day. Eva cherished the memory of Colin Powell – a lifelong supporter of Boys and Girls Clubs – sitting in the Kids' Kitchen with her kids and eating a pb&j.

Eva's Cute Soup

One winter I got the flu so bad that I went to bed and didn't get up for four days. Eva came to my house to take care of my kids and me. Of course, she wanted me to eat. I told her I didn't have the strength to chew. So, she made me soup with everything chopped so finely, I almost didn't have to bother. It was the cutest soup I'd ever seen. Every bit tiny and wonderful, just like Eva.

- One chicken, boiled, bones and skin removed
- Water from boiled chicken, saved and strained
° Onion
- Carrots
- Celery
- Peas – fresh or frozen
- Chicken fat
- Salt
- Pepper
- Dried parsley
- Chicken bouillon
- Cute pasta – alphabet or stars work great

Clearly this can be made (and in Eva's mind – should be made) with leftovers from a prior roast chicken dinner. But at the time I got sick, I didn't have any leftover chicken dinner and Eva made it from scratch. The key to cute soup is that every vegetable is finely chopped – to one quarter inch or so (the size of the peas or a little smaller). The chicken pieces can be – if necessary – slightly larger. Also, if Eva had a leftover chicken dinner, she would have saved the drippings and had plenty of chicken fat. Or a boiled chicken's broth, refrigerated, will also produce chicken fat for sautéing. Eva's mom – born in the first decade of the 20th century ALWAYS had a can of chicken fat in the fridge. She used it to cook everything! It was the fat that she used to make pie crust – which, now that you're asking, was delicious.

Finely chop all the vegetables except the peas. Sauté the vegetables in the chicken fat. Add water from boiled chicken (or drippings from leftover chicken and some hot water). Add bouillon and pepper to taste. You likely won't need salt if you use the bouillon. Add pasta and bring to a boil. When the pasta is cooked, the soup is ready.

Eva's Stuffed Apples

- Any variety large, tart apples
- Some sugar
- Some cinnamon
- Some raisins
- Some walnuts
- Butter

Eva did not use walnuts if she made these for the kids. She used the walnuts for me!

Peel and core as many apples as you have guests. Using your best judgement to evaluate the size of the opening left by coring the apple, in a bowl mix sugar, cinnamon, raisins and walnuts. Eva had special individual pans to make these. But you don't need that. All you need is aluminum foil. Tear off squares that will completely enfold one whole apple and butter the center of the shiny side. Set each apple into the center of its foil wrapper. Fill the hole with the sugar, cinnamon, raisin and nut mixture. Wrap foil up and close at the top. Bake in the oven at 350 degrees for 20 minutes (or longer if you like very mushy apples) and serve with ice cream (of course!)

Eva told every child she ever gave a ride home to that her car had a serious malfunction. She said that far beyond her ability to control it, her car pulled into ice cream parlors, and she simply couldn't stop it! Then she would drive by Dairy Queen or something – on purpose. If she was taking the child home, (as she often did for my kids when I worked late), she'd act surprised when the car would start pulling toward the driveway. She'd pretend that she was trying to stop the wheel from turning. It was adorable and every child fell for it.

I miss Eva, dearly.

Chapter Eight

Fundraisers, Church Suppers and Other Tribal Offerings

Central Pennsylvania's churches have a magnificent Easter tradition of making chocolate peanut butter eggs and selling them to raise money to help others. Nearly every shop in the community will have eggs for sale, for cash, with a steadily filling envelope of money going to fund the needs of others. The eggs are so delicious that eating them seems to be enough reward. Patrons needn't consider the fact that – in at least one case – the money raised provides shelter to persons experiencing homelessness in the town.

My favorite setting for the peanut butter egg sales is at the local saloon cash registers. Even though they compete with food sales, the eateries and drinkeries share valuable counterspace with these seasonal delicacies. Often, after a long session of drinking, the last purchase of the night will be an egg to sop up one's libations. The fact that the treat helps persons in need might even be lost on the willing customer as they soothe their cravings.

You'll find an excellent example of these delicacies on the following page!

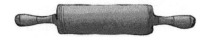

Jody West's Perishable Easter Eggs

She named them: Best Peanut Butter Eggs

- 1/2 c. butter
- 1/2 c. honey
- 1c. creamy peanut butter
- 1/2 c. 10x sugar
- 1/4 c. non-fat dry milk
- 16 oz bag chocolate chips
- Slab of paraffin
- Wax paper or parchment paper

Mix first five ingredients in order listed. Batter should be stiff enough to shape into eggs. Place on papered cookie sheet. Freeze until solid and ready for dipping.

Melt chocolate chips over double boiler.

Add 1/4 slab of paraffin (I just shaved some in.)

Stir occasionally until glossy.

Use two forks to dip eggs in, letting excess chocolate sauce fall back into bowl. Place on papered cookie sheet.

Makes about 20. Refrigerate or freeze until needed.

People getting together and publicly sharing food dates way back – to before the common era (BCE). Greeks, Romans and the early Jewish people all feasted in common areas. The Haggadah, a Jewish text, beckons, "All who are hungry come and eat."

In the holy month of Ramadan, members of Islam celebrate breaking their daily fast with communal meals known as Iftar. The Qur'an requires the faithful to feed others and promises that Allah rewards those who do.

Christian church potluck dinners, coupled with seasonal sales of everything from ribbon candy to hot cross buns, mean that people from different homes eat the same things at relatively the same time. Whether together in the church hall – or at home watching holiday specials on TV – fundraising food drives are another agent binding shared communities together.

Here are some dishes that friends have cooked at home and shared in their own communities. Through their recipes, they hope to share them with you.

Devera Lang's Tuna Casserole

- 1 - 10 1/2 oz can Campbell's condensed cream of mushroom (or cream of celery) soup
- 1/2 cup of milk
- 1 cup frozen (or canned, well drained) green peas (or mixed vegetables)
- 2 - 5 oz. cans of tuna packed in water (well drained)
- About 2 cups medium egg noodles (cooked and drained)
- 2 Tbs plain, dry breadcrumbs
- 1 Tbs butter melted

Preheat oven to 400 degrees F

Stir soup, milk, peas (or veggies), tuna, and noodles in 1 ½ quart casserole or baking dish. Bake 20 minutes or until hot, stir. Mix breadcrumbs and melted butter in a small bowl, sprinkle on top of casserole. Bake 5 min or until the breadcrumbs brown.

Pastor Chris' Funeral Potatoes

One of many side dishes or entrees traditionally prepared by church-goers for the funeral of another congregant. Chris calls it a classic midwestern casserole – full of cheesy, potato goodness.

- 1 large bag frozen shredded hash browns THAWED
- 2 cups sour cream
- 10.5 ounce can cream of chicken soup (or homemade)
- 10 Tablespoons butter, melted
- 1 teaspoon salt
- ¼ teaspoon freshly ground black pepper
- 1 teaspoon dried minced onion
- 2 cups shredded cheddar cheese
- 2 cups corn flakes cereal

Mix everything except one cup of cheese and all the cornflakes in a big-ass (technical pastor term, they assure me) casserole dish. Bake until gooey. Top with the reserved cheese and cornflakes, broil until golden and yummy-looking.

Kelly's Sweet and Sour Kielbasa

Not all potluck dinners need to be time consuming. The advent of jarred sauce and prepared foods (we get to this later in the book) changed millions of American lives. Kelly swears by this exceedingly

*simple recipe. Consider serving over rice, or just as an add-on at a
public supper.*

- Kielbasa
- Can chuck pineapple
- Jar maraschino cherries
- Jar duck sauce

Brown kielbasa in a large pot. Add everything else. Heat through.
Can be kept warm in a crock pot or in a chafing dish.

Lori's Traditional Passover Charoset

Friends since childhood, I reached out to Lori for one of her favorite
meals to share.

*"I cannot recall ever celebrating without food. Passover is a
particularly special event because it celebrates freedom." I'll let
Lori continue explaining in her own words. "Passover has several
meaningful foods that are used as symbolic for the Passover seder.
One is at the end of the Seder. We have a fruity, but bitter, Charoset.
Charoset is present on the Seder plate, representing the mortar
the Hebrews needed to work with during their enslavement. In the
Haggadah (prayer book for the Seder) it states, 'They embittered the
Jews' lives with hard labor in brick and mortar.'*

*"Additionally, it is made with sweet apples, for the sweetness of the
time. The bitter cinnamon in it represents the bricks that were made
for the pyramids in Egypt. This dish captures the symbol of slavery
and redemption of Passover."*

Traditional Charoset

- 3 medium apples, peeled, cored and finely diced
- 1 1/2 cups of walnuts, finely chopped
- 1/2 cup of sweet red wine, Manischewitz
- 1 1/2 tsp of ground cinnamon
- 1 Tbs. of brown sugar, packed
- pinch of salt

Chop everything up and add in a bowl all ingredients. Let sit for
several hours. Serve on Seder plate during Seder.

Marian's Award-Winning SPAM and Potato Bake

- 1 large onion, finely chopped

- ¼ cup margarine or butter
- 12 oz can low-sodium SPAM, thinly sliced
- 6 medium potatoes, boiled and cut into wedges
- 1 tbsp of dried parsley flakes
- 4 to 8 ounces grated shredded cheddar cheese
- 2/3 cup evaporated milk (or light cream)
- salt and pepper to taste

Melt half the butter in a pan and fry sliced ham until it begins to brown. Remove SPAM from pan and sauté onions until caramelized. Cut boiled potatoes into wedges and arrange in a two-quart baking dish with cooked onion and SPAM. Season with salt and pepper. Add evaporated milk; cover with grated cheese. Cover with foil and bake in pre-heated oven at 350 degrees F for 30 minutes. Uncover and brown in oven for 10 minutes longer. If you can't find low-sodium SPAM, follow the recipe and use zero added salt.

Dirt Dessert

This recipe inspires some creativity and is great for springtime holiday dinners. Makes an excellent centerpiece. "Kids love it!"

- Large plastic flowerpot
- Artificial flower (cover bottom of the stem with clean plastic wrap)
- 16 ounces cream cheese
- 3 cups milk
- 2 small boxes of pudding – any flavor you like
- 2 tsp vanilla
- 2 16-ounce containers of non-dairy dessert topping, thawed
- Package of dark chocolate sandwich cookies (think Oreos)
- Package gummy worms

Soften cream cheese and beat in a mixer for five minutes. Beat milk and pudding mix together until thick and add to cream cheese. Add vanilla – keep mixing. Fold in non-dairy topping. Crush entire package of cookies. If flowerpot has hole in the bottom put plastic wrap or wax paper inside. (You can also cut a disk of plastic from the bottom of the dessert topping container – for more support). Put half the cookie mixture on the bottom, then layer the pudding mixture – topping with rest of cookie mixture. Put in the refrigerator to chill. Before you serve, add gummy worms to "dirt" mixture and poke flower into the top.

Mickey's Homemade Beer Bread

Mickey worked in a Concord, New Hampshire food pantry and would make two dozen loaves for every fundraising Christmas fair. Everyone loved it and it her bread always sold out. This recipe calls for self-rising flour. If not available, use regular baking flour and add 1 tbsp of baking powder and 1 tsp of salt.

- 12 fluid ounce can or bottle beer
  (you can use club soda but it doesn't taste as good)
- 3 cups self-rising flour
- 3 tbsp white sugar

In a large bowl mix together sugar and flour. Add beer, continuing to mix, first using a wooden spoon, then your hands. Batter will be very sticky. Pour into 9 x 5 inch greased loaf pan. Bake at 350 degrees for 50 or 60 minutes. Tap on the top. Listen for hollow sound when done. Top will be crunchy; insides will be soft. Slice when cool and top with butter and jam. It also goes well with soup. *(Sadly, it's not good for sandwiches).*

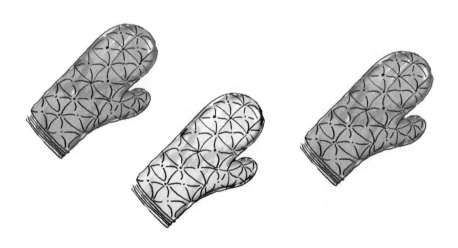

Blue Corn Bread

My son, John, sent me this recipe from Farmington, New Mexico, where he was teaching at Navajo Preparatory School. The whole family benefitted from his time there. I made one of my best new friendships, Maggie Deswood. Maggie's cooking is so delicious. Sadly, I can't duplicate her talents. I just must settle for relishing the meals we share together and appreciating how often she cooks for me and my family. You'll find this recipe calls for juniper ash. Not easy to come by outside the U.S. Four Corners area – but a vital part of the recipe.

Mix the following dry ingredients together.

- 2 cups Roasted blue cornmeal
- 2 cups Blue Bird flour
- 6 tablespoons Powdered buttermilk
- 1 cup Sugar
- 1 teaspoon Baking powder
- 6 tablespoons Juniper ash
- 1 teaspoon Baking soda
- 1 teaspoon Salt

Wet ingredients

- 1 stick butter
- 1 ½ cups water
- 2 eggs

Preheat oven to 400 Fahrenheit. Melt butter in a cast iron pan. Swish around. Beat eggs in a large bowl. Add the water. Dump dry ingredients into the bowl and whisk until combined. Add batter to cast iron pan and stir again. Bake for 20 minutes until middle has set.

Chapter Nine

WIC, SNAP & Other Well-Intentioned Humiliations

Food assistance in the United States began in 1939. The great depression of the twentieth century caused food surpluses. Farmers couldn't sell food because Americans didn't have the financial wherewithal to feed themselves and their families. Employed as a way to move the nations' farm excesses to dinner tables, the U.S. Department of Agriculture launched a stamp purchasing program.

People on "relief" – a term that dates back to the 15th century and connotes a level of want requiring public assistance – were allowed to buy $1.50 worth of food for just $1. The extra fifty cents could only be spent on surplus food – identified as such by the U.S. Department of Agriculture.

Clumsy and difficult for some people to use, the U.S. Congress tried for decades to create a program that better helped farmers and fed needy Americans. One night while campaigning in West Virginia, John Fitzgerald Kennedy promised hungry Appalachians that he would deliver a feeding/farming program, if elected. With his very first executive order, JFK did what no collection of lawmakers before him could do. February 2, 1961, he created the Food Stamp pilot programs. According to the Harvard Public Health Magazine, Kennedy's food stamp program helped 42 million American families.

Fast forward to the post Ronald Reagan war on the poor.

Disinformation during the 1980s blamed public ills on a fictional 'welfare mom' who schemed to rip off the American taxpayer.

On August 22, 1996, William Jefferson Clinton – perpetuating the myth that people receiving assistance were not worth the investment – signing the Personal Responsibility and Work Opportunity Reconciliation Act. He set into motion changes in the way economically disadvantaged people received necessities like food.

Cruelly, Clinton and his vice president bragged about shredding the economic safety net built by Roosevelt, Kennedy and Johnson.

Co-authored by then Ohio Congressman Mike Kasich, they added a sunset clause that eliminated food stamps (or Supplemental Nutrition as they came to call it) for everyone who was unemployed and not classified as disabled. Twenty years later, millions of people were impacted by their cruelty. In a case of ironic bad timing, the lost assistance caused great pain just as Kasich launched a Republican campaign for president. The last opponent standing at the end of the primary season, Kasich got trounced by a fast-food addict who would go on to serve Quarter Pounders in the White House. There's some poetry in that, but not enough to make up for all the pain they caused.

My book, Still Left Out in America, takes a deeper dive into the cruelty of this legislation. For now, I prefer to highlight the good work done when feeding our neighbors. In honor of JFK's fulfilled promise of food stamps to America's hungry, here's my mom's recipe for his favorite food – Fish Chowder.

Genevieve's Phenomenal Fish Chowder

In her early twenties, Genevieve and her girlfriends would rent a cottage for a few weekends each summer on Cape Cod in Massachusetts. One evening before either of them were married, she ran into JFK at a nightclub. I loved it when she told the story of dancing the night away with him. His romantic exploits were not then public, but I believed my mom when she told me that all they did was dance.

- Two large onions – sliced any way you want. (But I like big pieces of onion)
- ¼ lb butter
- ¼ lb salt pork (optional)
- 1 lb white fish, I prefer haddock or cod

- 2 large russet potatoes (more or less depending on your love of potatoes)
- Water
- Heavy Cream
- Salt and Pepper

Melt butter and sauté the onions until well cooked. Salt and pepper them liberally. I like lots of pepper in mine. Peel and cube the potatoes. Add to pot along with enough water to cover the chopped potatoes. Boil until the potatoes are cooked. Add the fish. It will break up while cooking. Boil roughly 10 minutes, then add cream – but do not boil after cream is added. Serve immediately.

WIC

The United States Department of Agriculture shoulders much of the responsibility for feeding America's most economically disadvantaged individuals. Depending on various income guidelines and other state-specific regulations, nearly twelve and a half percent, more than 41 million U.S. residents receive SNAP, the Supplemental Nutrition Assistance Program more commonly referred to by the name used for its predecessor, Food Stamps. Additionally, 2024 marks the fiftieth anniversary of a specifically created USDA feeding initiative known as WIC – the Special Supplemental Nutrition Program for *Women, Infants*, and *Children*. WIC provides targeted dietary supports to pregnant persons whose incomes fall below 185% of the poverty level, as well as their newborn babies and children through their fifth birthday.

Forty percent of all U.S. children, birth through four years of age, receive supplemental nutrition from WIC. That's an enormous number of kids in the wealthiest nation on earth getting nutritional supports based on family income.

The program provides funding for certain beneficial foods. Milk, cheese, cereal, vegetables and fruit. Five-year-olds who want to continue drinking milk, eating fresh vegetables and fruits or having a tasty block of cheese had better get a job when the WIC benefits end. I'm being facetious – but seriously, what's the point of ending a nutrient-specific feeding program just as a child starts kindergarten?

Steph Landis, a doula who makes her own soaps and salves to sell at local farmers' markets, gave me a recipe that she's eaten since she was a child. It's a family favorite that she makes for her own children. It uses ingredients moms can get on WIC and I thought this would be a nice time to share her recipe.

"This soup was a family favorite when I was growing up. Now that I am a single mom, with 3 kids of my own, I realize that this comfort food was made often because of its low cost. My mother stayed home with us while my dad worked construction jobs. Raising 3 kids on one income meant making a little bit go a long way. Cheese potato soup for the win! Since I've started making it for my own kids, I like to add fresh herbs like chives, thyme & rosemary. Sometimes, we get fancy and use Gouda cheese." (Serves 4)

Cheese Potato Soup

- 6 peeled potatoes
- Chunk of butter
- Few tablespoons flour
- Cup (or so) of milk
- Block sharp cheddar cheese
- Finely chopped onion

Boil potatoes in water until soft. Drain (but keep) the potato water. Make a roux in saucepan with butter and a few tablespoons of flour. Once paste-like, then add potato water to make a creamy sauce. Add milk to potatoes and mash.

Add to the roux/water mixture to give the soup desired consistency.

Cube sharp cheddar cheese in bite-size chunks to cover bottom of individual soup bowls.

Add salt and pepper to taste.

Pour hot liquid soup mixture over cheese and garnish with onion.

School Lunch

Turns out that poorly nourished, would-be soldiers got rejected when they attempted to enlist in the military during World War II. In response, not long after the war, Harry Truman signed the National School Lunch Act into law.

In 1966, Lyndon Johnson added breakfast to the school time benefit.

Over the years, the program has changed. Ronald Reagan tried to save some federal cash by slicing 1.5 billion 1980s dollars from the program. (That's 4.8 billion in today's dollars). Among his cost-saving initiatives: reclassifying ketchup as a vegetable.

Michelle Obama made short-lived improvements in the quality of the meals kids received. Subsequent elimination of the progress she made came under the afore-mentioned fast-food president.

If you interview kids, school lunches get mixed reviews. Although most of the kids I interacted with in the shelter voiced gratitude for a decent, often hot, meal.

Of late, the big scandal around the midday feeding of school kids is school lunch debt. According to the Education Data Initiative, in 2024, kids and their families had unpaid meal costs of $262 million with more than 30 million children owing an average of $180 dollars for the year.

Some states have addressed the problem in the most humane way possible. For example, in New Mexico, every kid is fed, every day, no questions asked. On the other hand, at the end of the 2024 school year, Pennsylvania had $80 million outstanding for school meals. I believe this is classified under states' rights. The right to have - Children. Owing money. For Lunch.

McKinney-Vento

One of the most remarkable and effective, problem-solving programs instituted by the federal government has to do with children experiencing homelessness. Early in this century, President George W. Bush pushed through signature legislation nicknamed, "No Child Left Behind." Universally deemed a drag on the education system by instituting testing requirements designed to rewire school funding, the program led to underfunded schools in poor neighborhoods. Still, there was one shining aspect to the law.

Before Bush's bill got passed and before he could sign it, a Republican congresswoman from suburban Chicago tacked on protections for kids without homes. The law provided for an expanded – and far more accurate – definition of homelessness, and it removed all barriers from education for unstably housed kids. This included *no questions asked* access to free lunch.

Back in 2011, I interviewed Congresswoman Judy Biggert following a trip to DC – activists were protesting in favor of more funding for housing. Diane Nilan (who knew Biggert personally) and I had testified in Congress about homelessness. Afterward, she gave me a few minutes for a story I was writing that ran in the *Huffington Post* later that week.

This brilliant woman, champion of educating kids experiencing homelessness, had just voted against HR 1 – aka the American Recovery and Reinvestment Act (ARRA). At that time, the ARRA was the single best legislation to provide for housing Americans since Johnson's multi-pronged war on poverty in his Great Society initiative.

I asked Biggert if she saw a contradiction between passing a mandate that all children experiencing homelessness receive assistance from school departments and then voting against funding housing initiatives that would help tens of thousands of kids. She said that she did not. I looked up the old HuffPo story and fished out the quote she gave me.

Biggert's response was, "there's going to be pain for everybody." Even though – moments earlier she'd said that schooling was "often the only source of stability and security" some kids have.

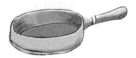

People are funny, aren't they?

Let's put aside the congresswoman's deeply rooted contradictions and return to the origins of her landmark legislation. In the early 2000s my traveling companion, Diane Nilan, worked with others – including Biggert – to craft her amendment to the bill and get it passed. Not surprisingly, Biggert's bill required no federal dollars. Every school department in the nation had been mandated to provide assistance to kids experiencing homelessness but the feds provided zero dollars to make that happen.

That initial, unfunded nature of the bill did not stop thousands of school departments from having top-notch liaisons. These education professionals are tasked with identifying children and youth experiencing homelessness, then helping them succeed.

One such champion is Salt Lake City's education specialist, Mike Harmon. This dude is so good at his job, he's been honored by local volunteer organizations and tapped for distinction by the U.S. Department of Education. Additionally, he makes things happen on the national scale with the National Education Association.   Recently, the Assistance League of Salt Lake City gave him an award for making sure that kids experiencing homelessness had clothes! Clothes! I could go off now on a discussion about the wealthiest nation on earth and school kids without clothes – but that would distract me from the task at hand – food!

Another great talent of Mike's is cooking. Diane and I crashed at his house on one of our tours – *Dismazed and Left Out*, we called it – and this generous man cooked for us.

Now, I'm a German Chocolate Cake fan. While there, Mike made a German Chocolate Pie – that was exquisite. When I got home from that trip, I made myself one. I was stunned at how easy it was to do. Mike told me he used to eat at a restaurant that made it. When they closed, he reverse-engineered a recipe so he could make it for himself.

Here's that recipe.

German Chocolate Pie

- 9" pie shell
- ¾ cup sugar
- 1/3 cup cornstarch
- ½ tsp salt
- 3 cups milk (2% or whole milk)
- 4 egg yolks slightly beaten
- 2 ounces German Chocolate (can use semi-sweet)
- 2 tablespoon butter
- 2 teaspoons vanilla
- ½ to 3/4 cup pecans
- ¾ cup coconut

Bake pie shell and set aside.

Mix sugar, corn starch and salt in a microwaveable bowl. Slowly add milk and mix well.

Microwave until mixture thickens and is at boiling, stirring frequently (typically 4-5 minutes). Continue cooking for approximately 1 minute. Slowly (very slowly unless you want scrambled eggs in your pie) add at least two cups of hot mixture into the egg yolks, mixing constantly, then add this mixture back into the large bowl and mix well.

Microwave for one-two additional minutes. Remove from microwave and add chocolate, butter, vanilla, pecans, and coconut. Mix well and pour into pie shell. Press plastic wrap onto top of filling.

Refrigerate for at least 2 hours. Remove plastic wrap when serving, and top with whip cream.

(Optional) I place a shallow layer of mini semi-sweet chocolate chips after the crust is cooked, but before the custard is added.

And, lest you think there's nothing savory in his repertoire, here's another recipe from Mike.

Chicken & Broccoli Casserole

- 20 oz. frozen broccoli (can use equivalent of fresh)
- 2 cups chicken, cooked and cubed into large size pieces (approx. 6 breasts)
- 2 cans of cream of chicken soup, undiluted
- 1 scant cup mayonnaise
- 2 Tbs. lemon juice
- ¾ cup soft breadcrumbs (I use buttered toast cut into small squares)
- ¾ cup grated cheese

Prepare broccoli according to directions or steam fresh broccoli, and place on the bottom of a 9 x 13" greased baking dish. Next place cooked chicken on top of broccoli. Mix soup, mayonnaise and lemon juice in a medium mixing bowl, and place on top of chicken. Place the breadcrumbs then sprinkle cheese on top.

Bake at 350 degrees for 30 minutes or until bubbly. Also delicious with leftover turkey.

Chapter Ten

Inflation

On April 12, 2022, the feds announced the U.S. inflation rate exceeded eight percent – the highest increase in more than forty years. The prior twenty-six months of a deadly, global pandemic caused the American worker to re-evaluate the value of selling their labor on the cheap. Generous U.S. federal unemployment compensation to workers who lost their jobs when the country shut down allowed individuals to select carefully the route they employed when rejoining the work force. Wages leapt upward.

Round after round of stimulus funds coupled with a year of dependent child subsidies had returned much of the cash to the market that had been lost when businesses, schools, churches and agencies shuttered their doors to stave off anticipated pandemic death tolls.

Sadly, the American people approached pandemic precautions as haphazardly as they do most things. Splitting down political lines, science deniers, anti-vaxxers and self-proclaimed freedom fighters succumbed to their illnesses in record numbers.

A year of lockdowns kept Americans home and off the road. Oil companies lost money and blue skies shown over cities in India for the first time in years.

When Covid19 protocols relaxed, people retook to the roads. Fuel prices climbed to pre-pandemic numbers and just kept going. Then, on

February 24, 2022, Russia invaded her neighbor, Ukraine. Europe's largest fuel supplier clobbered the world's largest supplier of low-cost wheat. Fuel and food prices skyrocketed as a stunned first world slapped sanctions on the aggressor, shutting down Russia's oil and gas exports to the west. At the same time, the third world reeled from a loss of desperately needed cooking oil and grain.

On the morning of April 22, National Public Radio (NPR) aired a news package complete with interviews of impoverished families discussing their inability to make ends meet. As a journalist, I get irritated by news stories that miss the point – a point of their own making!

The people interviewed – one from a family of two trying to survive on $1600 each month, and another woman incapable of saving a security deposit and forced to live in a fleabag motel – discussed their plight. What was NPR implying? That eight percent increases even mattered in the general scheme of things to families and individuals too poor to survive even if the prices had not increased at all?

Want my definition of middle-class? A middle-class person can buy fresh cherries without looking at the price. Poor people don't buy cherries. As Christie reminded me when I interviewed her for this book, buying any fresh fruit at all – even on sale – is just too much of a gamble. What if it spoiled?

I've taken children living in homelessness to baseball games and other events with tickets donated by a local Rotary Club, and the kids don't even ask for a hot dog or to stop for fast food – because they've never done it. They don't have a frame of reference for such consumer behaviors.

Sure, inflation hurts the middle class, but real poverty isn't even phased by a twelve-dollar steak increasing to a cost of twelve-dollars and ninety-six cents because they weren't buying that steak in the first place.

Seriously – I have given spare change needing to be counted to a kid experiencing homelessness and the child didn't know a dime from a nickel. There is poverty so severe in the United States – so desperately in need of correction – that inflation due to corporate greed or a mild uptick in wages can't even touch it. According to a 2024 report by Market Watch, one half of the American people are under water. A companion piece on CNBC says that 44% of Americans wouldn't have a way to tackle an unexpected $1000 expense. ONE HALF of Americans owe more than they are worth. Literally, if you put two random people from the U.S. in a room – only one of them would have more assets than debt.

Inflation is a problem that plagues those who can already afford fresh fruit, transportation costs and rent. Millions of Americans languish in abject poverty, a topic seldom discussed and therefore never rectified. Food insecurity isn't about, "Oh shucks, darn, that's more expensive." It's about, "We were on assistance before and now assistance doesn't even cut it."

Tonya Zuber – a poet I met because she was doing poetry slams about homelessness – explained to me how inflation is affecting her family. One of their favorite cheap meals isn't cheap enough anymore. She's got a grammar school-aged daughter, a high school-aged son and herself to feed. When the pandemic ravaged America (and the world) the feds doubled everyone's SNAP benefits. Without that extra allowance, Tonya and the kids are in deep trouble at the end of every single month.

Here's a recipe for one of their favorite cheap meals. It was easy to make at the homeless shelter's shared kitchen, because it didn't take long to prepare. But now she can't afford to buy the canned beef stew anymore. Corporate greed drove the price of a can of stew from three dollars each to more than eight. And this recipe calls for two cans. So, the small family doesn't eat it anymore.

Tonya's Family Favorite Beef Stew

"This meal is $21.45 assuming you already have milk, butter and eggs at home."

- 2 38 oz cans of Dinty Moore Beef Stew
- 1 packet McCormick Beef Stew seasoning
- 5 lb bag of potatoes
- 1 box Jiffy cornbread mix

Empty both cans into a pot along with the seasoning packet. Fill one of the cans a little over half full of water and add it to the pot. Stir it while it heats. Make mashed potatoes and cornbread. When everything is done, pour the beef stew over the top of the mashed potatoes and serve with a slice of cornbread. It's yummy and filling!

Tonya's Family Favorite Mashed Potatoes

"If you're doing it to be cheap – leave out the cream cheese."

- 5 lb bag of potatoes
- Stick of butter
- 8 oz brick of cream cheese
- Salt and Pepper

Peel, slice and boil potatoes. Mash with stick of butter and brick of cream cheese. Salt and pepper to taste.

Tonya's Fried Cabbage and Kielbasa

- 1 head green cabbage
- 2 lb. package of kielbas

One last gift from Tonya – the poet. BTW – you can find her on TikTok talking about the issues that plague real people. She took time, while sharing her family recipes, to mention that she'd been inspired by Humble Pie and created a poem for you. Here it is.

From Those Who Are Hungry

Do you know how it feels to go without food
To feel the hunger gnaw at your stomach
As your head's pleading
While you're daydreaming
About what it is you could be eating
Do you have to choose to pay the electric
Or have a bite to eat
I know it's a constant struggle
A never-ending defeat
The prices of food
Are outrageous beyond belief
Food is not a luxury
It's a necessity for relief
Most are house poor
Making just enough to survive
Leaving most without much
Barely staying alive
It's a harsh reality
A cruel punishment
When you're forced to go days without a meal
Or any real nourishment

Food banks are overwhelmed
And resources are stretched thin
Families are still starving
Now how's that a win
Searching for good potatoes
In a bag of ones that are old
Drinking milk past expiration
And eating bread that has mold
We're just supposed to be thankful
For the food that we are given
Knowing damn well they wouldn't consume it
If they were in our position
Families expected to survive
On canned meat and food that's outdated
Don't complain
Be grateful
If you're hungry you will eat it
Our system is broken
Those in power turn a blind eye
To the suffering
To the pain
To the tears the people cry
The cycle of poverty
It's a never-ending fight
For families are expected to survive
On scraps and leftovers each night
People plead for help
For understanding and accommodation
Only to be met with ignorance, neglect and frustration
No one should go hungry
In a world of abundance
Yet far too many are left to suffer
In silence and reluctance
It is time for those in power
To open their eyes and see
And deal with this major issue
They call FOOD INSECURITY

Now it's 2024, and inflation is easing. But the impacts of those initial price hikes have left a mark. Low-income eaters need to eat differently.

Once-inexpensive canned meats must be replaced. If they have a way to cook, they can eat beans. Beans are healthier and much cheaper. Bags of dried beans are the cheapest – but few food banks supply slow cookers.

Betsy Garrold, a messaging specialist who represents farmers at the state and federal level, has a message for those agencies that distribute free foodstuffs. "If you're gonna give out dried beans, you better be giving out crock pots, too." Eating less expensively is labor intensive. And most low-wage earners work a lot of hours to make ends meet.

Beans are great for low-income vegetarians, especially. But the added vegetables needed to make a bean dish tastier can get very expensive. In Carlisle, our local farmers' market offers two market bucks for every EBT (food stamp) dollar spent – generously making fresh vegetables more affordable to SNAP recipients in my town.

In honor of the Farmers on the Square, I'm leaving you with my favorite vegetarian chili recipe. It would be vegan, but when I serve it, I sprinkle it with cheese. Your call on that – cheese ain't free. This recipe also calls for fresh vegetables – also not free. I hope you enjoy making it. And just for fun – try making it by using only canned veggies and see if it still passes muster.

Vegan Chili

- Olive oil
- One zucchini
- One summer squash
- Green pepper
- Fresh jalapenos (1/2 cup chopped)
- Brightly-colored peppers
- One onion (two if they're small)
- One pound of chopped spinach or kale
- Two large cans diced tomatoes
- Two cans of red kidney beans or black beans or one of each
- Ground red pepper
- Ground black pepper
- Chili powder
- Ground cumin
- Rice
- Cheese if you want to break out of the vegan and go straight-up vegetarian.

Chop all the veggies into bite sized pieces and sauté them in oil. When tender, add canned tomatoes (Fresh tomatoes work, too, but I seldom have enough fresh tomatoes to use them so liberally). Add spices to your liking. Generally, a teaspoon of everything except just half a teaspoon of cumin. Simmer over medium heat. Pour cans of beans into a strainer and rinse until they stop making bubbles. Add to the chili. Cook enough rice for everyone and serve with chili on top, then sprinkle with cheese. They do make vegan cheese but that too is expensive. Idealism is costly and most folks must give up non-violent lifestyle choices when they are poor. Which makes sense, because poverty is violence.

Remember to try this again using only canned vegetables. Sweet potato would be tasty but mushy, I imagine. Yuck for the rest of what's available in tin.

Now try to make it without a stove or access to running water.

Poverty complicates everything.

Chapter Eleven

Food as a Weapon

Many federal agencies are tasked with addressing the needs of the poor. The food program often referred to as Food Stamps, now called SNAP (Supplemental Nutrition Assistance Program), falls under the supervision of the U.S. Department of Agriculture. TANF (Temporary Aid to Needy Families), once thought of as "Welfare," is a block grant program that many states play political games with – often causing even more hardship.

In many states, only a tiny fraction of those in need get help. In the early 2020s, Pennsylvania, one of the greatest offenders, siphoned off 89 percent of TANF monies, sending funds instead to agencies like anti-abortion religious groups. Consequently, Pennsylvania helps remarkably few children and their families with the remaining eleven percent.

Newly elected officials, including Governor Josh Shapiro – in cooperation with the first-ever Black woman elected to be Pennsylvania's Speaker of the House, Joanna McClinton – are working to redirect this funding. Progress is slow because of the stranglehold their opposition has on the PA senate – coupled with the fact that neither of them has completed a full term in their respective offices. Time will tell if they can redirect TANF monies to families. And that's just one state. Nationwide, only twenty percent of TANF funds (according to the Center on Budget and Policy Priorities report dated September 23, 2024) actually go to families who desperately need the funds.

One of the agencies most commonly associated with poverty, HUD (the U.S. Department of Housing and Urban Development), does a whole lot more than provide an ever-dwindling amount of housing opportunities to an ever-growing number of poor people. As was revealed during the Donald Trump administration – when his son-in-law was famously flagged for taking millions in HUD monies to fund his burgeoning New York real-estate empire and bilk the poor. HUD also oversees the highly popular middle class mortgage tax deduction, which is the largest housing investment for individuals and families HUD has. The middle-class mortgage tax credit doesn't just fund a family or individual's primary residence, but a second home as well.

The average American more likely believes that Section-8 housing – private landlord compensation for renting to low-income individuals, or public housing developments funded in part by the feds and owned by local housing authorities – consumes the lion's share of tax dollars for housing. But they're wrong. The middle-class mortgage incentive costs American taxpayers far more. A stinging truth for those experiencing homelessness but paying income and sales taxes – finding out that their dollars are used to pay banks for mortgages that they themselves are too poor to access.

There are other agencies – in addition to the Department of Agriculture – Health and Human Services, the Department of Education, the Federal Emergency Management Agency and more. But, for the sake of this book's focus on food insecurity and in honor of a kind woman who agreed to share her story, we'll stick to HUD.

Karen Eckrich grew up in an abusive home. That's germane only because HUD cares a lot about domestic violence. HUD has very narrow definitions of homelessness and very little interest in the personal lives of people experiencing homelessness. (Think none).

The agency claims to keep count of folks experiencing homelessness, and the tally they keep is based entirely on quantifying the number of abjectly marginalized individuals with zero resources. Because of HUD's penchant for counting people who are visibly on the street or in a shelter, their methodology limits the Point in Time (PIT) count almost exclusively to folks with problems so large that being seen is the least of their concerns. (Think addicts and folks with mental illness so severe that they can be observed on street corners, under bridges and in abandoned parking lots). Added to that is the total number of shelter residents reported to the agency by overnight missions and other emergency shelter providers.

When HUD identifies these easy-to-find folks, the questionnaires generally focus on three basic categories: Are you or have you ever been a victim of domestic violence? Are you a U.S. veteran? Are you HIV positive? If the person answers yes to any of these questions, they may jump the line of folks waiting for housing.

For decades, HUD ascribed a vulnerability quotient – the VQ – which assigned a numeric rating to a person's misery. The agency tries to be a little less outwardly macabre now, but they prioritize wretchedness all the same. Knowing that hundreds of thousands of people struggle with chronic illness, addictions, mental illnesses, not to mention the fear that their abuser might finally locate them, doesn't entice Congress to allocate any more funding. When dispensing housing vouchers, there literally aren't any more funds directed to house these people, once identified. This tragic lot just get preferred status to the other persons experiencing homelessness who do not fit into one of these categories or refuse to be counted and consequently the misery numbers are pitifully low.

But, back to Karen.

Poverty and hunger made Karen's childhood less than ideal. There are many stories (I've got a few in this book) that tell of hungry families that navigate the challenges before them with love and courage. But those stories are more often told because they suit the needs of the reader. The stories of poverty setting the stage for hunger, homelessness, conflict, and abuse are difficult to consume. So, they remain concealed. Karen courageously allowed me to share her story with you.

Karen's dad, a bully and an alcoholic, would hunt or fish for the family's daily meals. He hunted with a shotgun because buckshot was more affordable than bullets. Karen described it this way, "It was expensive to hunt. It still is. He even tried making his own bullets for a while, but that, too, was more than he could afford. Deer hunting was better. He'd hunt with a bow and arrow. But we had squirrel and rabbit a lot more often than we had deer."

Karen remembers chewing squirrel or rabbit meat carefully so she wouldn't crash her teeth down on buckshot pellets. One day her dad told Karen's mom to look in the basement for breakfast. He'd brought home a basin of freshly caught fish. When the young girl and her mother went down cellar, they found his catch and knew, "If we wanted to eat, we had to kill them."

Even as a young child, Karen got very adept at killing and cleaning her own food. "I can clean fish really fast because I don't like to do it. But I'm good at it." Her dad cleaned the small animals he shot. "Daddy would clean the game. I got the bunny tails." Killing and gutting animals to feed a family is a noble act, unless it's done by a sadist who uses feeding the family as a way to terrorize his family.

Not riddled with backward-facing blame, Karen has come to understand the poverty dynamics that made her father (and her mother) who they were. "Daddy was a warped young man who went to WWII. My mom didn't really know what she was doing. God help us, they got married when Daddy was only seventeen."

Like most meals, wild game and fresh fish tasted better with vegetables, in a stew or as a side dish. Karen was grateful when there were vegetables in the back yard to add to their menu. "My mom had a small garden. She grew tomatoes and onions. But mostly she grew flowers. We had a lot more flowers than food."

I have a friend named Candy. Her dad punished her by withholding food. He didn't employ a go-to-bed-without supper kind of discipline. He preferred the go-hungry-any-time-of-the-day-or-night sort of torment. Unsure of what would set her father off, Candy would squirrel away balled-up slices of white bread to eat when her dad would deprive her of food for particularly long stretches. On top of that, when not on restriction, she was lactose intolerant and often the food she was forced to eat – like free government cheese – made her sick.

During our interview, I mentioned the irony of a food bully naming his child after a sweet treat. A charming, polite woman her mid-fifties, Candy replied, "Fuck! I never thought of that."

Politicians use food as a weapon too. Most recently, famously and tragically – Russian Prime Minister Vladimir Putin and Israeli Prime Minister Benjamin Netanyahu. A quick web search reveals the atrocities committed by both men, who've excused their actions as the consequences and necessities of waging war.

The United States has famously built a landing platform for humanitarian aid brought to Gaza by the sea – a colossally inadequate solution to a Netanyahu-created problem. Putin has expanded his war to include the weaponization of exports. The Ukraine supplies – or did before February of 2022 – foodstuffs to impoverished African nations who have become casualties of the Russian oligarch's lust for power. Putin cut off exports from Ukraine's sprawling breadbasket/farmland to the starving nations to their south. You literally don't have to take my word for it – I've included references to some decent journalism on the topics in the bibliography.

Of course, ruthless tyrants don't just run other countries. Here in the U.S., in the summer of 2024, the federal government extended a pandemic-era policy supplying supplemental nutrition dollars through Department of Education-identified families by augmenting their SNAP allotments. But fourteen governors turned the money back – refusing to help kids in poverty receive improved access to food.

The reasons given by Republican governors across the nation varied from inadequate computer processing capacity to a philosophical opposition to the concept of welfare. While the well-fed grownups in those fourteen statehouses bickered over theoretical dependency, kids with genuine hunger pangs went unfed.

My friend, Matthew Best – a Lutheran minister who cares deeply for people and we work together on lots of projects – says that the cruelty is the point. It's not about upgrading software or instilling expectations of entitlement in five-year-olds. It's about being cruel and deriving satisfaction from all that power. The power to deprive children.

Oh, by the way, of the fourteen, Nebraska finally relented and fed their hungry kids. Go Nebraska!

But seriously, that deserves praise?

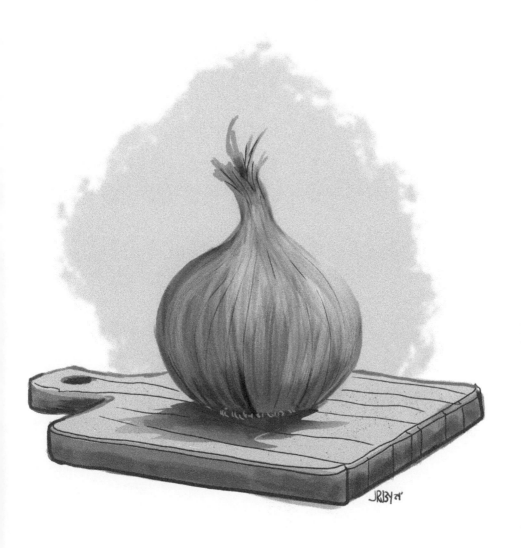

Go Your Own Way

Chapter Twelve

Dooryard Delicacies

Foraging, some people call it. And if you've ever taken to the woods in early spring – perhaps looking for hardwoods and hunting a batch of Morel mushrooms growing by their trunks, then you know exactly what foraging is.

When I interviewed Momo Mass – a refugee from the Democratic Republic of Congo – she lamented just a few things that she'd had to leave behind when she fled her country. Most importantly, she hated leaving her mom. But secondly, she missed, "public food supplies."

Momo explained to me that most food came from other countries – think the aforementioned shipments from Ukraine to Africa. In August of 2024, Africa News ran a story detailing "devastating social upheaval" because of food shortages caused by the war in Ukraine. Momo told me that the politics of the DRC, "doesn't really promote agriculture," but that the fruit bearing trees were public property.

Occasionally in the U.S., you'll hear of a community planting edible plants in public. In fact, the U.S. Department of Agriculture has an Urban Fruit for Urban Communities project that you or your town council might want to explore. (Yeah, the link's in the bibliography).

To Momo's point, most fruits and vegetables growing in the United States are private property. Walking into an orchard or farm and plucking something to eat is a really bad idea. You don't have to take my word for it – just ask Beatrix Potter's friend Peter Rabbit.

If you're one of those Morel mushroom hunters – unless you have a nice forest or apple orchard of your own - you're likely trespassing to grab your dinner. Public food supplies versus ownership of that food has been a problem since before the Magna Carta was written in 1215 and issued at Runnymede in a place that used to be called England.

As a matter of fact, public access to food was one of the biggest reasons the Magna Carta was written. Nobility – from the king down to the lowliest lord – owned everything. Hungry peasants hunting rabbits were trespassers and thieves, and the punishment could be fierce. Not to get too far into the weeds on this – hungry serfs who worked the land for their landed masters often had too little to eat. The elderly, widows and orphans, without anyone to work the land for them, had nothing. Until the Magna Carta!

Fearful that the starving masses would overthrow the feudal system of the time, King John – portrayed in Disney cartoons as an immature and cowardly lion – agreed to apportion some of nature's more public resources to feed the peasants. One could draw a ragged line from the Magna Carta to the social programs of today. Why should the wealthy own all the food? Why shouldn't a portion of the world's bounty go to folks less fortunate?

I'll leave you to mull that over and get back to the topic at hand – folks who forage.

I loved interviewing people for this book. Each person I spoke to had a different story and I have the honor of emphasizing why their story mattered.

One afternoon, I joined a three-way call with my friend Chris and their mom, Rose. After a few cursory instructions like, "Turn the volume up on the side of the phone, Ma," we got started.

Rose came from a huge family. She shared a recipe for "bean soup" that, far as I could tell, almost never contained beans. My mom called her version of the creation garbage soup. I can see why people would prefer to eat Rose's soup if they based their decision on the name alone.

"Mom died when I was five years old," Rose explained to me. Her dad remarried and they moved to a farm in Kentucky. Her stepmom was a good cook. The farm had fresh vegetables and between her stepmom and grandmom, "there was always something in the skillet."

These women made their own sausage – Goetta – a way to stretch limited amounts of meat by mixing it with oatmeal. Rose loved Goetta fried with eggs.

Because they lived off the land, Rose and her siblings (there were nine of them under the age of thirteen) didn't always have as much as they'd like to eat. But, she reassured, "we wasn't sickly."

The family didn't have individual birthdays. There were just too many of them to celebrate, so the clan would have one big party, once a year.

In addition to what they could grow intentionally, the land around their home provided lots of tasty morsels. Dandelions, rhubarb, honey from bees and, of course, mushrooms. Any delicacies they ate depended on the season. (I'm personally ecstatic when I see a patch of rhubarb growing wild and often dismayed when I see it sold in the grocery store for more than $5 a pound).

Rose has fond memories of the foods she ate – especially the results of their home canning that preserved the fruits and vegetables grown on their farm.

Chris cherishes the skillet handed down from her grandmother – the one that was never empty. And, knowing Chris, I'm sure it's not empty now.

Looking back on her childhood, Rose waxes philosophical about living off the land, "I might not have had what I wanted, but I never went hungry."

Here are a few of Rose and Chris's family recipes.

Dandelion fritters

"Dandelion fritters. I remember my great-grandma Elliot making this."

Pick dandelion flowers. Rinse them and only keep the heads. Throw them in a Ziploc bag with a little bit of cornstarch and shake it until they are covered. Make a batter with cornstarch and milk and black pepper and salt. Dredge the dandelions in the batter and throw them in hot oil.

"I actually want to try this again this spring. I remember liking them when I was little."

Fiddleheads – a northern clime variation of gathered dandelions –

grow abundantly in the springtime in places like Maine. I journey there often, and Chris constantly reminds me to stop on the side of the road and harvest some of these wild ferns which are among her favorites. Fiddleheads can be made into soups and sauces, but Chris usually just sautés them in butter or olive oil and serves them hot with salt and pepper for seasoning.

Beans and Cow Soup

Cow soup or Bean soup – it was often called either. This was different literally every time. You take whatever meat ends you have - a little leftover chicken, piece of meatloaf, hot dogs, whatever, and if it isn't enough to make another whole meal, you put it in the freezer in a big Ziploc bag. Same with little bits of vegetables. I generally keep them in two separate bags. And when the bags are full, you defrost them and chuck the contents of the meat bag and the vegetable bag into a big soup pot and let it simmer until you have soup. Add the odds and ends of dry pasta you have in the pantry at the very end of cooking.

Chris cautioned, "At the outset, once you take the bags from the freezer, you might want to sauté the vegetables first then add the meat and continue from there."

Vinegar Pie

Pie Crust (there are several recipes elsewhere in this book)
- 4 eggs
- 1 cup light brown sugar
- 1/4 teaspoon kosher salt
- 6 teaspoons melted butter
- 2 teaspoons apple cider vinegar

Make a pie crust – don't cook it. Then whisk the eggs, brown sugar, apple cider vinegar, melted butter, and salt together. Pour into the pie crust. Bake in a hot oven until set. Grandma's "Hot Oven" is 375 degrees

Water Pie

Good and Deep Pie Crust
- 1 1/2 cups tap water (Grandma said, "boil and let it cool, if you have a well.")
- 4 tbsp flour

- 1 cup white sugar
- 1/2 teaspoon salt
- 2 teaspoon vanilla
- 1 teaspoon cinnamon
- 5 teaspoons butter in thin slices off the stick

Make a good, deep pie crust, then pour the water in the unbaked pie crust. Mix together the flour, sugar, cinnamon, and salt in a bowl. Sprinkle it over the water in the pie crust. DO NOT STIR IT. Make sure it's even, but let it settle itself. Drizzle the vanilla over the flour mix, and lay the slices of butter over the surface of the pie.

Put it in a 400-degree oven for 30 minutes. Then reduce to 375 and cook 30 more minutes. It's gonna look raw when you take it out. Let it set on the sill until it's cooled off, then stick it in the icebox. It'll set up in the icebox.

(Grandma called the refrigerator an ice box because when she was a girl they kept things cool with ice.)

Grandma Elliot's Carrot Cake

- 2 1/2 cups flour
- 1 cup white sugar
- 1 cup dark brown sugar
- 1 1/2 teaspoon baking soda
- 1 teaspoon baking powder
- 1 teaspoon salt
- 2 teaspoon cinnamon
- 1/2 teaspoon nutmeg
- 1 cup melted Crisco
- 1/2 cup melted butter
- 4 eggs
- 1 teaspoon vanilla
- 3 cups grated carrots
- 1 cup chopped black walnuts
- 1/4 cup bourbon

Mix everything together but the bourbon. Pour into two greased and floured cake pans. Bake in a hot oven until your testin' stick comes out clean. Put your bourbon in a glass and set it on fire so the alcohol burns off (or don't, if you want a little hooch in the cake – for adults only). Poke some holes in your cake layers with a toothpick. Pour the bourbon over the layers. Frost with cream cheese or vanilla frosting.

Chris didn't give me her grandma's frosting recipe. I make my vanilla frosting with room temp butter and – when I have it – cream. Milk works fine but doesn't taste as rich. My secret ingredient is marshmallow fluff – any brand will do.

Butter Cream Frosting

- 8-ounce stick of butter – brought to room temperature
- 12 ounces powdered sugar (more or less)
- 1.5 teaspoons vanilla
- Some cream (or milk)
- Generous serving spoon scoop of marshmallow fluff.

Cream the butter in the bowl with the back of a spoon. If you have a mixer, you can just mix on low for a minute or so. Add powdered sugar (with a mixer, this can get to be an airborne mess – perhaps go to the spoon for the initial mixing). Add the vanilla and perhaps a little less than a quarter cup of milk or cream. If you make it too wet, add more powdered sugar.

Once the frosting is the correct consistency, stir in the marshmallow fluff. If you'd prefer chocolate frosting (although maybe not for carrot cake) just add a 1/2 cup or so of unsweetened cocoa powder BEFORE you add the marshmallow fluff. The fluff should always go in last.

Hunting and the law

When we first moved to Maine, my dad – then a newly minted chief of pediatrics – started a rural pediatric outreach. The hospital where he worked purchased a full-sized camper van and then decked it out like a mobile clinic.

Allagash, Maine – a miniscule town in a monstrously large county – had existed for decades – centuries even – relatively untouched by the outside world. The community was so isolated from the rest of North America that Allagash residents of the mid-twentieth century presented a rare genetic disorder caused by intermarriage. My father, in addition to being a kid-doctor, specialized in genetics. He regularly traveled into Aroostook County, to Allagash and other hamlets to provide healthcare and conduct genetic research.

My dad was two men. An empath when looking out at the world, and nearly pitiless at home. Paul had grown up in a tough household. With a bully for a father, and little disposable income, he muscled his way around the neighborhood and school.

His time in the military netted him a college education – thanks to a post-World War II, fully funded, GI Bill. From there he attended medical school and vastly improved the socio-economic prospects for himself and his family. When he saw others face adversity, he felt deeply for them. When someone in my house had it rough, we needed to put up, shut up and remember how lucky we were to have a roof over our heads and food in our bellies. A "Stop crying or I'll give you something to cry about" kinda guy at home.

Not long after he started that pediatric outreach, my dad traveled into "the county" and down the long logging roads to Allagash. He regularly visited a family that hadn't left the region in generations. Justifiably, the rugged individualism of woodsmen who lived off the land impressed my dad. He loved it. He admired the family and got to know them well. (It didn't hurt that their genetic anomalies afforded him the opportunity to study rare hereditary conditions).

One week, my father returned from the Maine woods, completely shattered. He wept openly for a man he'd met up there. An Aroostook dad had ventured onto public lands and shot a moose. His family had little food and hadn't eaten regularly in weeks. In the dead of winter, five-hundred pounds of moose meat would fix that problem – for a long time.

By the early 20th century, hunters had slaughtered the moose herd to near extinction. In 1935 the legislature banned the practice of moose hunting entirely. My father's encounter with the hunter and his family happened in 1976 – four years before wildlife biologists declared the herd rebuilt and a citizen's referendum would legalize the practice. The hunter my father met went to jail. Ill-gotten spoils, the authorities confiscated the meat. The family's hunger persisted.

I have a feeling my dad bought the hunter's kids some groceries. I sure hope he did. He'd done things like that in the past. At the time, he was so upset, I hadn't thought to ask.

I didn't have a recipe for moose from my high school days. But the following recipe is from the The Salvation Army in Waterville, Maine. Officers from the corps prepared this dish during the big ice storm of 1998. Much of the northeast from New England to the Canadian provinces was powerless for nearly a month and 34 people died. Lots of people – especially those who ran soup kitchens – struggled to cook the food that spilled from their rapidly defrosting freezers.

Waterville Corps Moose Stew

- 3 pounds moose meat
- 7 cups beef broth
- 3 yellow onions
- 2 cups chopped celery
- 5 potatoes
- 3 large carrots, sliced or chopped
- 6 cloves garlic

8 1/2 stick butter

- 1 tablespoon salt
- 2 tablespoons pepper
- 1 tablespoon chili powder
- 3 tablespoons cornstarch
- Fresh rosemary and thyme tied in a bundle

Cut your moose into bite-sized chunks (perhaps one-inch cubes) and, using some of the butter, brown off with salt and pepper. Slice your onion and cook until soft in some of the butter. Throw your onions, moose, celery, carrots, garlic, butter, the rest of your salt and pepper, chili powder, rosemary and thyme bundle into a pot with the beef broth. Bring to a boil and reduce to simmer. Simmer until everything is tender. Cube and fry your potatoes in the rest of the butter. Coat cooked potatoes in cornstarch and throw them [along with the rest of the cornstarch] into the pot. Cook until the broth is thickened into gravy. Add more salt and pepper to taste.

I don't know who called for so much salt, but if using salted broth, I would scale back on it considerably. Moose is gamey, which could be the reason for salting it so heavily, but my blood pressure went up just typing this recipe.

Chapter Thirteen

Grow Your Own

According to the University of Michigan's Center for Sustainable Systems, more than 83% of Americans live in urban settings. Want to know why people think more people experiencing homelessness live in the cities? Because more people experiencing anything live in cities. Fewer rural unhoused people? Sure. But fewer people in general. The point is, poverty combined with trying to feed yourself and your family, sucks – everywhere – it's just easier to hide in the countryside. Turns out, hunger is also easier to cure there.

Rural patches of land, coupled with a few seeds, may yield foods that offset the less- nutritious groceries available to the financially disadvantaged. What 1970's rural kid doesn't know someone who dropped a few marijuana seeds in the woods and grew their own supply?

That same idea works for food. This is different from foraging. This is planned growing and harvesting on land leased to you – or – on someone else's land. And, while not well-studied, it's likely as common as living in an abandoned warehouse or taking shelter in someone's seasonal home. End of discussion.

We don't have numbers, but if you own a piece of land in part of the American rural expanse, you might consider contacting local outreach workers (I prefer homeless liaisons in the schools – they know what kids are in need) and offering a patch to folks in need.

Perhaps – if you're not into lending use of the land outright – you can work a deal where you get a portion of the harvest. Or better yet, let a young person use it on the condition that they share the produce with an older person living in poverty. That way your generosity helps two people at once.

Lending your land has far-reaching benefits. Rural, suburban and urban farming doesn't just provide more stable access to nutrition – it helps the community in general. Monique Allen, in an article written for The Garden Continuum, listed six great reasons to grow your own food. From pesticide reduction to reduced carbon emissions, growing your groceries makes sense. These truths aren't such great incentives for the financially disadvantaged who haven't the luxury of worrying about tomorrow's impact of today's actions. (Literally – they don't – if you'd like to argue that point, call my publisher and I'll visit your local library where we can have a lively debate).

From Allen's list, the best motivation for the poor to grow their own food is improved nutrition. Another of her reasons, improved flavor, also fills an immediate need. But where do those on modest budgets get a piece of urban ground to till? Or the time to cultivate it? Short of you donating a piece of your land?

Everywhere you see flowers growing publicly – for the benefit of everyone – that's a spot where vegetables or fruits might do the same. And you may be aware that some towns have public gardens. Most charge a fee to rent and till a parcel of land.

In the waning days of the last century, my kids and I lived in affordable housing. We lived in a town outside Portland, Maine where elevated housing costs made low-income renting impossible without help. Some of us in that Freeport development paid our own rent without subsidy, but the local housing authority kept the cost of our places below market rate and, therefore, affordable.

An Afghan family lived three units down from ours. The dad had been a professor in their home country. If you remember your history, Russia occupied the nation from 1979 thru 1989 – and the coincidental war left Afghanistan in tatters. That was before the U.S. invaded 12 years later. I can't imagine what's left of the nation now.

At any rate, I don't know the details about why this highly educated, English speaker and his family fled to the U.S., but there they were – in Freeport, Maine – and they adapted the best they could.

The father worked as a hospital interpreter – not a great paying job. His three children excelled in the local public school system. His wife, Latifa, spoke zero English, and I spoke zero Dari or Pashto. Against these odds, we became friends. We mostly used sign language to communicate. We'd point to magazine photos or objects in our houses to explain our thoughts. Eventually I came to understand her needs. I could help her with some of them. Like the day that I drove her to a job interview with local retail giant, LL Bean, where she got a job sewing.

One day she brought a picture of a farm to me. Then, she walked me to a plot of land about a half mile away where I learned that Freeport had a public garden. Her paycheck, not hers to spend, went to the family. I quickly figured out that she didn't have the cash to rent the land or buy the seeds.

A journalist, working as a part time bartender, I told all my customers about this woman. I explained that she needed cash to get a little patch going. One of my regulars gave me thirty dollars. The next day I used half of it to rent a plot of land in the public garden and took her shopping with the other half. She purchased seeds.

Honestly, after that, I forgot all about her little enterprise. I never went back over there. She continued to work full time mending tents or replacing zippers or doing whatever it is that LL Bean seamstresses do. After we did the paperwork to rent her space, I never gave her another ride to the plot. If she had gardening tools, I never saw them.

One day, a few months later, she knocked at my door with a bowl full of vegetables. Latifa's harvest had begun! Every week that fall she knocked at my door with "my share" of that week's produce. She fed both our families with 60 square feet of land and a $30 dollar investment. I can't assign a dollar figure to her labor. I hear folks enjoy gardening. I hope she did.

Could helping people like my Afghan refugee friend have their own gardens fill a nutritional need in this country? Of course it could. And – according to *The Garden Continuum* – it could reduce carbon emissions & pesticide use, reconnect us with nature, teach us about our environment and even improve the flavor of our meals.

How does this story end? Well, a few months later my mom died. She left me enough money for a down payment on a small house. We didn't need public housing anymore. We moved away. You'd think this story would end "and I never saw Latifa again." But it doesn't.

Every Saturday that I went to the local farmers' market, I saw her. She hadn't just grown food for her family. With me gone, she took her abundance of veggies and started a business. She cooked for others out of her home with the produce she'd cultivated. She learned to speak English, fluently. Her kids graduated and went to good universities. Industrious and hardworking, she eventually left LL Bean and cooks now, full time.

Years later I moved out of the area. I might've thought that I'd never see Latifa again, but I heard from her one last time. Several years into the new century, when the license for her home kitchen needed renewal, she called me. The state of Maine had a backlog, and they would not inspect her operation until months after her license expired – effectively putting her out of business.

Even failed politicians have connections. (You likely don't know about my political exploits. That's how ill-fated they were). I called mine and they adjusted the inspection schedule, moving her up the list. It had been an oversight, one that she could not get corrected on her own. At some point in time everyone needs a little help – even the most self-sufficient among us – a fact many choose to ignore.

A week later I heard a knock at the door. There stood my friend, Latifa, holding a plate of onion naan dripping with olive oil. She'd traveled 50 miles to bring it to me. My share of the license, she said.

Onion Naan also known as Naan Pyazi
(Explained by Latifa, but Americanized by me)

- 3 cups flour
- Some olive oil (maybe ¼ cup)
- Some salt
- Start with a cup of water
- Cooking oil
- Stuffing for the bread
- Onions – five or more chopped finely
- Salt, pepper & oil to sauté (You can use whatever fat you enjoy. Butter, even).

Sauté onions in oil with salt and pepper.

In a bowl mix water, salt and oil – add flour to make dough – set aside for 10 or 15 minutes.

Make dough into a ball then roll it out with a rolling pin. Or flatten with your hands. Latifa used her hands to make just about everything. Spread the flattened dough with onions to lightly cover. Roll the dough over onto itself, like a tube. Then coil it around itself and flatten with your hands.

Heat very thin layer of cooking oil in pan. Place coiled pressed bread into the pan and spoon a small amount of oil onto top. Allow to cook a few minutes then flip and cook the other side.

Latifa would serve this with a spoonful of onion/olive oil mixture on top as a tasty addition. But if serving with other saucy things, you might want to omit that part.

Obviously – for the more adventuresome cook – the sky's the limit on what to do/add to this recipe.

Other home farmers grow what they can in anything from window boxes to five-gallon drums filled with soil. Here are a few more recipes for those who get an abundance of fresh veggies from the most meager of patches. My friend Jody grew up with access to a small parcel of land and a great big beautiful cherry tree in the back yard. (She's the one who makes the peanut butter eggs featured earlier in this book).

Too Many Tomatoes in the Garden Pasta
Tomatoes and Macaroni

- 5 fresh tomatoes or two of the largest cans of canned tomatoes
- 1/2 C. of any dry macaroni or small pasta
  (bowties, elbows, etc.)
- Sugar to taste (Try 3 tablespoons, stir, then taste. Add more sugar if necessary.)

Boil pasta according to pkg. directions. Drain. Return to saucepan. For ease of peeling, dip tomatoes into a separate pot of boiling water. Add tomatoes and sugar to cooked pasta. Simmer until heated through. Spoon into bowls. Eat with crackers or buttered bread/rolls.

"Look on day-old shelves in grocery stores. The bread is usually pretty fresh. Margarine or oleo (oleomargarine was the original name of the plant-based spread. In the 1950's and 60's it was often called oleo for short) are OK too. Or serve with grilled cheese sandwiches."

This recipe can be adjusted to feed more people. It's different from mac'n'cheese – a tasty, filling way to use up the last garden tomatoes. Guess you could also add basil, but my mother didn't use herbs.

PS. A former neighbor made "buttered noodles" for her day-care kids by cooking the pasta, adding butter or oleo and a dash of salt. And giving apple slices or other seasonal fruit for lunch.

Cherry Pie

"Not sure that the Cherry Cobbler is a recipe for Humble Pie. For us, yes, because the cherries were free. Anyway, to the best of my knowledge, the recipe follows:"

- 3 c. Bing (dark, sweet cherries), fresh (Don't know, but frozen might work too)
- 1/4–1/2 c. sugar
- Dash of salt
- 1/4 tablespoon cornstarch
- 1/8 teaspoon almond flavoring (Optional—I prefer it w/o the almond)

Mix fruit and dry ingredients together, stir then pour into pie or square pan. Add crust to top. Cook 30 min. at 350 degrees.

3 to 1 Crust

- 3/4 c. flour
- 1/4 c. solid Crisco shortening
- Pinch of salt
- 3-4 tablespoons cold water (or more)

Blend Crisco into flour until it looks pebbly; add pinch salt. Add enough water to make a smooth ball. Roll or flatten crust with rolling pin, rolling from center out until you have an 8"-10" circle. Place gently on top of cherry mixture. Cut a 'C', star, or other symbol in center for steam to escape. Or cut crust in 1/2" lengths and weave them into a lattice.

"PS. May need more sugar—but cherries are pretty sweet. Enjoy with whipped or ice cream."

Chapter Fourteen

Stealing

My grandson, Ronan, and I have written a couple of books together. They're science fiction/fantasy novels with a social justice bend. The stories are all Ronan's. He wanted to support the kids that he knew went to his school – who were just like him – except that they didn't have homes. My daughter suggested that Ronan dictate the stories to me and that I write them in a chapter book form. The *Kursid Kids* series – the third is due out in 2026 – is artfully illustrated by Aron Rook.

For the most part, my job was similar to Aron's. She turned chapters into pictures after I'd turned Ronan's concepts into paragraphs. Ronan's so imaginative that I couldn't have improved on his creations of a scientist, a sentient robot and a genetically modified magic cat – even if I'd tried. But, one time, thinking I better understood our audience, I attempted to change one of his fundamental concepts. During one of our Zoom sessions, when Ronan would review my prose, I read him the altered chapter. Suffice to say, the child was not pleased. Our conversation went something like this:

"Grummy (my grandkids call me Grummy), I told you that the dad steals to feed his family."

"I know you did Ronan, but I thought giving him a low-wage, menial job that would fund their needs might make him more sympathetic to the reader. We don't want readers to dislike your characters because they steal."

"No, Grummy, you're making apologies for people who have no food. They shouldn't have to apologize. The wealthy who have more of everything than they need, much more than they could ever need, they are the ones who should be sorry."

Ronan was right. I stand corrected. Golden toilets when people have no spinach isn't the fault of the people lacking spinach.

And besides that, it's the Magna Carta, all over again. Who said the powers-that-be have a right to everything? Well, the powers-that-be said so. Duh.

Over the course of time, when the peasants threatened to become the powers-that-be, the nobility generally gave up enough of their wealth to quell the anger and unrest. Remember that in 1215, the peasants demanded that King John allow them to hunt and gather on royal lands. Afraid the villagers would deploy their superior numbers, the king relented.

Fast forward nearly a thousand years and *hangry* is the new-age term. It's a combo of hunger and angry – the former causing the latter. But hanger is nothing new. Like the Magna Carta, it has fueled revolution from the beginning of recorded history. Even George W. Bush, at the time of his 2008 banking crisis and subsequent economic collapse, knew enough to increase access to food stamps.

I explain all of this for one reason – to lay the factual groundwork that people steal to survive. If we can acknowledge that stigmatizing the thief is foolhardy, perhaps we can respect people who resort to law-breaking in a world that starves them.

The book of Proverbs from the Christian Bible states that, (and if you're curious, I'm using the Good News translation here), "People don't despise a thief if he steals food when he is hungry." That's not just what Ronan told me, that's from a two-thousand-year-old tome!

Or perhaps you'd prefer something from a more contemporary novel? How about Jean Valjean from *Les Misérables*? Published in 1862 by Victor Hugo, Valjean is incarcerated for stealing bread. But the author wanted to make a larger point. Knowing that his protagonist would need more than a morsel or two to survive, Hugo sets up a wealth disparity dynamic. Upon his release, the author sends Valjean to a church to be fed by a kindly prelate. When the hero finds himself surrounded by opulence, Hugo has him steal some ornate candlesticks. Upon discovery of the offence, Valjean's host, Bishop Myriel, gives the silver to the thief and hides his crime from the police. Myriel's generosity protects Valjean from further prosecution and provides him with ample resources to get back on his feet.

Still, understanding hunger isn't enough. Victor Hugo and my grandson both agree that understanding the desperation driven by hunger is essential. Let moral judgements be damned!

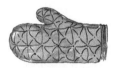

In September of 2011, a few hundred protestors took to New York City's Zuccotti Park and started a movement that would spread around the globe. Occupy Wall Street gave way to Occupy Melbourne, Occupy Montreal, Occupy Rome, Occupy Tokyo, Occupy Lima, Occupy Cairo and thousands of other cities, towns and hamlets across all six inhabited continents.

Critics of the tent villages that popped up, casting stark contrast to neighboring wealth centers, claimed that the organizers had no plan. A rather typical response from folks whose comfortable lives had been insulated from an economic downturn caused by the greatest financial crisis in nearly a hundred years.

In 2008, the Bush/Cheney economy collapsed when the housing bubble they encouraged crooked lenders to inflate, had burst. Eager for new leadership, voters elected the Obama/Biden administration to remedy the mess. A massive government bailout rescued banks, brokerage firms and insurance companies while everyday people lost their homes, jobs and often their life's savings. By 2011, the unemployment rate had crept within striking distance of 10 percent. One in 11 people were out of work, and the national mood felt desperate as everyday people learned that CEOs received bonuses for navigating a storm of their own making.

The Occupy movement became the clarion call for individual frustrations in the face of 2008's congressional corporate protectionism. Life in a nation where banks and financial institutions were deemed *too big to fail*, but ordinary workers felt their government had deemed them too small to save, just wasn't working for millions who'd been thrown out of their work and their homes. While the American Recovery and Reinvestment Act (ARRA), passed the following year, and even though it targeted many of the problems created when the economy collapsed, the ARRA certainly would have been more successful had all the money that went to members of the financial industry – like Bank of America's $45 billion bailout – gone to ordinary Americans instead.

Meanwhile, in a mid-sized city of the American deep south, Tom Garner suffered, living hand-to-mouth, in homelessness.

There are countless stories of people experiencing homelessness being welcomed into the Occupy camps. My own book, *Still Left Out in America*, contains a story about the Occupy Harrisburg group saving a local man's life. Tom – who blogs under the pseudonym, Gnat – is not the star of one of those local rescue stories. No Occupy camp saved him. And now, nearly 14 years later, he's still struggling to save himself.

In 2011, Tom had been living on the street, hunting for necessities and surviving inclement weather by sneaking in and out of a local church.

A smart man who was (and is) more than a little bit angry about the U.S. class structure that guarantees a constant supply of individuals and families will go without the barest of necessities, Tom founded Occupy Homeless. Much like the people he represents, his creation has no geographic home.

After learning about the protests popping up across the nation, Tom started an online Facebook community that is now populated by 10,000 residents. Additionally, he's started a companion Occupy Homeless Facebook group where hundreds of people share their stories.

I've interviewed Tom several times. He's a great source of unvarnished truth. And he's free with many of the facts of life that most people on the street prefer not to share.

As a self-proclaimed cynic who has seen way too much suffering, one of my favorites is his description of dumpster diving. Tom says, "It's not eating from the trash – it's eating trash."

Take a minute – let that sink in a little.

"I'm not happy to admit that I ate trash," Tom told me. "I did it because I had no choice. I have to admit that I'm more unhappy from being so low that I had to." And it didn't always go well. "I got sick from it [eating garbage], from time to time."

Dumpster diving and stealing food aren't new. Throughout time, humans have tried to make a "living" from what other people throw away. Tom explained to me that back in the Great Depression of the 20th century, "Hobos would collect garbage cans for people. Empty them. Wash out the cans and return them." They did this so that they could go through the trash and salvage what was palatable. "They ate from the garbage pails. And after they washed the cans, they called the rinsings, *Hobo Soup*."

Tom shared a modern-day recipe for Hobo Soup. I'll quote him here, again. "You need some stolen ketchup and/or mustard packets. Salt and pepper if you can find it. Then beg for some free hot water. They'll usually give you that."

Tom added that a person could make a real treat if they could get their hands on barbeque sauce packets to spice up the soup. "It's tough to steal the packets on your own. If you can get an accomplice, she could distract the clerk while you stole the packets."

Sighing, Tom added, "When I think of how many times [before homelessness] that the person at McDonald's gave me too many packets and I'd already driven away. So, I threw them in the trash. Now I think, *I was throwing away somebody's meal*."

One last thought that Tom wanted me to leave with you. It's not easy to launch an online protest forum with 10,000 members, like he did with Occupy Homeless. Mostly because it's often impossible to keep your laptop or phone safe from the elements. "When you 'live' in a wet and moldy environment, the used equipment doesn't last long..."

Not everyone stealing food to survive is an impoverished single white man with a massive online following. Nope, some of the other million or so underfed are people like Mavie.

As a teenager, Mavie and her family lived in their car. A lifestyle so precarious it resulted in lifelong physical disabilities as well as arrests for stealing trash. Yeah, you read that right. Turns out it's against the law to steal someone else's trash just because you think something in it might be worthwhile.

Because Mavie wrote to me about her experiences, I needn't attempt to transcribe an interview. You can read firsthand, like I did, the horror she experienced.

For me homelessness resulted in a major trauma. It was beyond scary living out of our car, getting shot at and people trying to break in and steal from us. We got to the lowest of lows and often talked of killing ourselves to not have to stay in the situation.

We were treated like less than dirt at the churches we went to, where, at most, I was asking for prayers to try and lift my soul. Sadly, I had the doors shut in my face.

Homelessness is getting so desperate that you take food from the dumpster. It's ignoring your own needs to help others around you, because you know what it's like to not have enough to survive, and to hurt.

Hell, I'm still more than willing to give the clothes off my back to someone else.

Homelessness is injuring yourself, because it's a free-ish night in a hospital, where you can get a few hours of rest.

Homelessness is giving away your dignity, because that's what organizations will require just to give you a meal.

Being homeless is usually not a choice but a situation that is forced on you. You will fight and struggle to get out of it. And most won't succeed.

I knew a father who would bike 10 miles, one way, just to get to work. He'd had to sell their car off. All because his wife died.

For me, it was a sick mom who lost her job. My brother left to go live with our sister, and everything piled up against us. I was only 19 when all of this took place. I was working 3 jobs trying to make us float a little bit and killing myself in the process. One of my employers even tried to scam me out of hours. I got blood clots in my legs from living in the car with my mom, but I couldn't just leave her there.

My main go-to as far as food was McDonald's. We would get the two-for-one burger deal. Mom would have one of them and I'd get the other with just bread and cheese. I'd get the meat on the side, which we would feed to our animals. It wasn't much, but it fed us for a bit.

If you went behind Walmart after they dumped the main food, you could get bread that had some mold spots. We'd cut them out. You could get milk that just expired and was kinda still OK. Squished bananas and overripe fruits were plentiful, but you needed to be careful.

One time we found frozen burritos, which I had pulled out. That's when security caught me. They called the police. I was crying. I couldn't get arrested because I needed to care for my mom. They let me drive to the station rather than leave mom alone. My autistic crying doesn't translate well. They took some pity on me. I mean, Mom was dying, and they said I wasn't a flight risk. But they still made me pay a $1000 fine for it.

It's been years now since Mavie lived in the car. Her mom is long gone but Mavie still has trouble caused by the thrombosis in her legs. She's trying to process all she went through. Therapy is helping. She summed it up this way, "My husband came home from the therapist one day, saying that he found a new allegory for poverty. It's a never-ending game of *Would You Rather*. The game descends steadily downward with increasingly sucky choices."

Food Not Bombs

I've known for decades that people get arrested for stealing food from dumpsters. I still can't type that without shaking my head about how stupid the notion is.

During my 2004 campaign for Vice President, I met a volunteer with a feeding charity called *Food Not Bombs*. I'll put a link in the bibliography. I've interviewed the founder, Keith McHenry, many times – both on the radio and for print articles I've written. He's a real American hero. *Food Not Bombs* salvages food and gives it to hungry people. Hardened criminals – the lot of them.

When our campaign visited Knoxville, Tennessee during the VP *Left Out Tour* – the trip that led to my first book on homelessness – one of the election volunteers who'd arranged my visit nearly missed the event. He'd just gotten out of jail – arrested for taking bagels from a dumpster.

Some Folks Just Don't Eat at All

As we know – not everyone who is hungry is homeless. Here's one more anecdote from a friend a couple of decades older than me who remembers experiencing hunger throughout her childhood. All recipes she thought of sharing from her youth involve a can, a can opener and lots and lots of ketchup.

Born into poverty, in Maine, in the 1940s, Susan remembered that no matter how awful the meal was, they couldn't leave the table until they'd finished every bite. She remembered her mom sitting in the parlor while Susan and her siblings ate.

It was generally something out of a can and utterly revolting. We would drench it in ketchup – tomato gravy. It was often canned hash. It bears no resemblance to my homemade corn beef, potato, and onion hash. As kids we would drown it in catsup and had to sit at the table until it was gone. I didn't realize then that my mother sat in the other room because there was not enough to go around. We thought she was getting away from the nasty food."

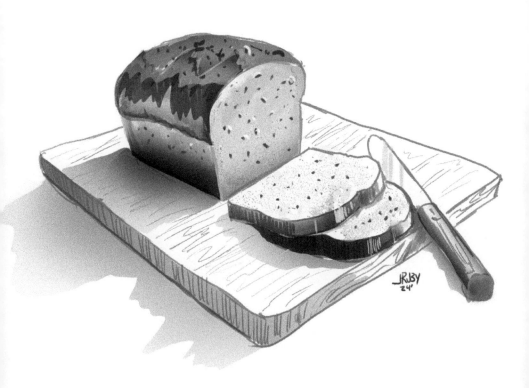

Innovation

Chapter Fifteen

The Pandemic

There's a great book, entitled *Pandemic 1918*, written by Catherine Arnold. It's a collection of eyewitness accounts from the influenza pandemic that ravaged the globe more than a century ago. It's been less than four years since our own once-in-a-century infectious disease catastrophe and two of my books already include references to the deadly coronavirus. I have no doubt that, for decades to come, the stories of our own pandemic will keep surfacing with nearly every phenomenon of the Covid Era chronicled in one way or another.

Since 2020, our diets, our practice of preparing food, certainly changed. Personally, my husband and I ate very little meat during the lockdown. Once the news broke that corporate meat packing plants refused to shutter their doors, resulting in widespread infection among the workers with subsequent alarmingly high death rates, we stopped buying meat. We also saved money – exchanging our restaurant tabs for grocery bills.

One singularity that I didn't participate in was bread baking. It's estimated (or rumored, or both) that someone in more than 40 percent of American homes attempted to bake their own bread at least once during the shutdown. *Eater.com*, an online magazine for foodies and other domestic types, estimates that while a fine loaf of sourdough bread might cost $10 at the bakery, home cooks can whip up the same crusty yumminess for about $2. With grocery prices on the rise, baking and eating one's own bread can be a treat for the wallet as well as a nice accompaniment for a pot of beef stew.

My son-in-law – along with millions of others – got caught up in this craze. Tim used the sourdough sensation to get in touch with his Belarussian roots. A newly minted U.S. citizen, Tim missed plenty about his homeland – not least of which was a dark rye sourdough bread called borodinsky. Week after week my son-in-law baked a new batch and with each iteration his product more closely matched the flavor he'd remembered from his childhood.

Mail-order everything also became a trend during the pandemic, and the self-taught baker started ordering his flour from Germany – so that his bread would be fashioned from grains more genetically similar to the ones back home. Consequently, your version of his recipe may not taste exactly the way his does.

Eventually, Tim achieved perfection and started shipping his bread to family members around the country so that we could have a taste of his youth. As you remember, we were all shut away from each other. I felt lonesome and missed my family. In some way, it better connected me to my son-in-law, who – even without a pandemic – had to wait years to see his loved ones because they lived half a world away.

During the pandemic, Tim's Priority Mail packages thrilled us all. We knew that inside the red, white and blue packaging, we'd find a loaf of his homemade bread. I particularly enjoy a slice of it toasted, with cream cheese. But you do you.

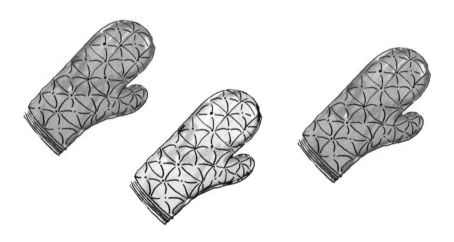

Tim's Borodinsky bread

"The key thing to remember - making this bread is not exact science, but rather a creative process. Because we are dealing with live sourdough bacteria, all times listed below will vary based on room temperature and humidity."

Stage 1: Prep the rye sourdough levain

This assumes you already have rye sourdough starter living in your fridge.

Before going to bed, mix 50g of rye sourdough starter, 50g of warm tap water and 50g rye flour. Cover with tinfoil or plastic wrap with some holes for breathing. Let sit overnight at room temperature. By morning, the levain should rise and be very bubbly. What you want to look for is for the top surface of the levain to start dropping a little.

Stage 2: Prep what I call "pre-dough"

You'll need:

- 33g rye malt
- 3 tsp freshly ground coriander
- 75g rye flour
- 250g very hot tap water (I heat it on the stove to 195 F)

Also, before bed, grind/blend rye malt and coriander. In a bowl, mix all dry ingredients, add hot water, stir well, cover with plastic wrap (again with breathing holes), wrap the bowl in a thick towel or blanket and let sit overnight.

Stage 3: prep the dough

You'll need:

- All of levain
- All of pre-dough
- 125g whole wheat flour
- 125g rye flour
- 47g molasses
- 1 tsp salt
- 50g very hot water

The next morning, in a large bowl add hot water, salt and molasses, mix well. Mix in levain. Add pre-dough and mix well. Add all flour and mix well. Cover the bowl with plastic wrap (with holes – the plastic always should have breathing holes) and let sit for one hour.

In the meantime, prep baking pan by lining it with parchment paper. With wet hands, take the dough out of the bowl and place it into the baking pan. Make sure to spread the dough so that it sits flat in the pan. Sprinkle with whole coriander seeds (coarsely ground seeds can work too). Gently press the seeds into the dough. Place the pan into a plastic bag with some holes in it and let sit at room temperature away from direct sunlight for several hours. In my case, I typically wait about 9 hours, although I've also waited as long as 12. But it can also take less time, depending on your room temperature. The idea is to allow the bread to rise just the right amount. You know that the bread is ready for baking when it has doubled in size and the top has formed a few holes. If the top looks like it's dropped, you've waited too long. I typically monitor this process throughout the day, and by evening I'm ready to bake.

Stage 4: bake the bread (note that ovens vary, so feel free to experiment with temperature and baking time)

Preheat oven to 550F, with a pan of boiling water on bottom.

Place baking pan with bread in the oven. Immediately lower to 500F and bake for 20 minutes. Take water out, lower to 400F and bake for 1 hour.

Remove the pan from the oven, take the bread out of the pan, remove parchment paper (sometimes it sticks) and let sit on a cooling rack for an hour or two.

After all this - enjoy!

Chapter Sixteen

The Omnipresent Onion

My mom went to college at the same time that I attended high school. I ended up doing a lot of her homework with her. I didn't do it for her – she always did her own work. But she didn't like to do it alone.

Pretty much everyone in my family has a gift for cyphering. Even the kids that didn't like math could do it. Genevieve, having dropped out of high school during World War II grew up believing she had no aptitude, but all she needed was a good teacher and a math buddy who had faith in her. We'd do her core class assignments together. I had fun. I think she did, too. After decades of putting yourself second to your husband's career, third to the needs of your children or dead last to the male-dominated world around you, it's great to have someone believe in you.

Genevieve's preliminary classes allowed her to dabble in biology and several other sciences. A huge fan of reading, she had to step away from her Agatha Christie novels to read a number of the classics. If she read a book, she'd get me to read the book, too. Then we would discuss it. I'll never forget the day she put Emile Zola's *Germinal* into my hands.

Originally published in 1885, a generation and a half after Hugo's *Les Miserables*, Zola echoes the message of resistance, but his coal miners are far less individualistic than Valjean and his contemporaries. The pro-union messaging in the book teaches the reader that Etienne, the protagonist, is saved by the social contract – something much less random than finding a generous bishop with silver candlesticks.

You already know what I'm going to tell you next. As much as the horrible working and living conditions of the mines fueled the rebellion in Zola's novel – starvation was the root cause of the mine strike and subsequent reforms.

I remember, as a 16-year-old kid, reading about the food scarcity the miners experienced. My heart broke when they exhausted their most important staple – the onion.

I remember asking my mom how people could survive on a diet of onions. I think back now – to my grandmother's origin story – and realize that my mom knew, all too well, the answer to my question. She told me, "For those people, onions were a gift." Followed up with, "You'd be surprised what you'd eat if you were starving."

It is surmised that humans cultivated onions before any other vegetable. One report I read, entitled *Onion History*, published by the National Onion Association (NOA) asserts that the first onions grown by farmers date back 7000 years. Those first onion farms were likely planted in a region somewhere between Iran and Pakistan. Pre-historic people moved from gathering wild food to planting their own – and that journey began with the onion.

As for the U.S.? Even though the Mayflower's manifest includes onions, that's not their North American origin. The Native Americans had already been cultivating them for millennia.

Here is my favorite onion soup recipe. I make my own version of French Onion Soup – it has so much more than onion in it. I'm sure I'm cheating. And yes, after I've prepared the soup, I get myself a nice crusty white bread and some gruyere cheese and place a bowl of the finished soup under the broiler with the bread and cheese layered on top. It's delicious.

You can find more onion recipes at the end of the book. There, my buddy Chef Archie and a few other professional cooks are featured. You'll find a copy of his tomato, onion and paprika soup as well as a butter baby onion recipe that's quite yummy, too.

Chunky Onion Soup

- Beef soup bones
- 2 tablespoons Better Than Bouillon Roast Beef Base
- (You can get some other brand of broth starter, but no. Don't do it).
- 8 or so Vidalia onions (any onions will do)
- Minced clove of garlic
- 1 lb. chuck roast cut into cubes (any cut of meat will do because you'll cook it for hours)
- 1 stick of butter
- ¼ cup flour
- ½ teaspoon salt
- 2 teaspoons pepper
- Half gallon of water
- Bay leaf

Boil the beef bones with the bay leaf in the water for five or so hours. Sauté the onions and garlic in the butter. Combine the flour, salt and pepper. Coat the cubed beef in the flour and brown the sides of the cubed meat in the butter and onion mixture. Dump the contents of the frying pan and the Better Than Bouillon into the stew pot. You can pull the bones out first or leave them in there to cook for another three hours. After a full day of cooking – voila!

Chapter Seventeen

La Sauce est Tout– The Sauce is Everything

In the latter half of the 20th century, the 1950's slogan of the Franco-American canned food company, *La Sauce Est Tout*, along with the French flag on the label, were used to advertise products that most consumers considered of Italian derivation. The company's introduction of pasta in a can – and later the infamous Spaghetti-Os product (which was easier to eat and designed for kids) – happened long after Campbell's Soup purchased Franco-American in 1915.

Originally, French immigrant Alphonse Biardot opened a Jersey City, New Jersey commercial kitchen with his two sons in 1886. At that point, he and his family had lived just six years in the U.S., having emigrated from France.

Not yet in the spaghetti business, a 19th century advertisement for Franco-American hawked, "French Soups, Game and Chicken Pâté." And, though the family sold the company less than 30 years later, Campbell's still uses the Franco-American label for sauces and gravies in their expansive product line.

I'm of French heritage on my father's side. Perhaps if my parents hadn't hated each other, I might have known more about what that meant culturally. My French grandparents, horrified when my dad brought home an Irish girl, shunned my mom and tried to talk my father out of marrying her. Knowing how their relationship would deteriorate, it undoubtedly would've saved them both a world of problems had they listened.

But then, you and I would never have met.

My dad's family lived on the *wrong side of the tracks*. Euphemistically, this term indicated an opinion by the well-to-do that the LaMarches were of low-class breeding and possessed a generally undesirable nature. My grandfather, a Boston mounted policeman, bullied people with ease. As a child I remember looking at his *billy club* (a wooden baton used by police to beat suspects and/or rabble-rousers) as well as his handcuffs, with dread.

In those days, lots of immigrants became cops. In the 1910s, 20s and 30s the job required few skills. Hormisdas, my grandfather, emigrated to the United States from Canada in 1905. Born in 1896, he married Eva – a daughter of Canadians who immigrated to Vermont, presumably to work in the brickyards.

By all accounts, life for the economically disadvantaged in 19th century Quebec rivaled that of similar European peasant existences. North American lumber barons replaced earlier royal masters continuing a legacy of hardship for the underclass. Woodsmen working in the great north forest barely eked out a living. Some grew crops when they could. Frigid winters made for short growing seasons. Few farmers could survive without moonlighting as lumberjacks. Late 19th and early 20th century Canadians of French ancestry migrated south to work in U.S.'s booming industrial regions.

As noted earlier, my dad's parents didn't approve of my mom's ethnic background. Even though early industrial America persecuted both the Irish and French for their Catholic faith, my LaMarche grandparents considered themselves superior to any and all Irishmen. This is significant for two reasons.

One – we should consider historic antagonisms when thinking of the horizontal hostility between ethnic groups in the 21st century. Why do poor American whites feel threatened by working-class immigrants? Could it be as simple as human nature? Primates when overcrowded will attack others of their species.

Two – it explains why my mother, the keeper of the home, preserved virtually none of my father's cultural history or family traditions – save one. French Meat Pie!

Let me share one last story before we examine the Franco-American gastronomical wonder known to others as Tourtière. By the way, we never called it that. My dad didn't, either. His French-speaking parents wouldn't teach their language to him or to us. More immigrant self-loathing, no doubt.

My mom maintained my dad's French-Canadian Christmas Eve tradition even though she despised him. Maybe she'd developed a taste for the meat pie before her tastebuds soured on him. As one of the younger children, I missed out on the part of their relationship where they cared about each other. Perhaps she started preparing the holiday specialty for him before I came along – at a time when my older siblings and cousins allege that she liked the man.

Allow me to share one of her regular comments about their marriage. Mind you, one of my mom's favorite sayings was *Many a Truth is Said in Jest*. Genevieve liked to recount, "The church your father and I were married in burned to the ground the very next day so that no other such unpardonable sin could be committed there, ever again."

I laugh thinking about it. It's true. The church did burn to the ground the next day. Still, I frown when I remember all the prejudice my Franco-American grandparents harbored against my mom. Their resentment of her ethnicity guaranteed that I would grow up knowing nothing about their ways and habits – except that they were cruel. What I know about the one custom my family retained from my dad's side of the family, I gleaned from research referenced with the other sources in the bibliography of this book.

Tourtière is a descendent of meat pies made thousands of years ago by the Greeks. Many versions of the double-crusted, shallow pastry, filled with assorted meats, became a staple in the Middle Ages. By the time the Franco-Americans created their version to celebrate Christmas, the recipe often included pork mixed with game. Early chefs chopped the meat finely. Now ground meats are used. The internet is filled with recipes for the tourtière that use fowl, rabbit or some other wild game. Along the way, cooks added potatoes to the mix.

The use of aromatic spices differentiates French Meat Pie (or, as my mom called it, Irish French Meat Pie), from similar dishes. For years people speculated that the use of cinnamon or clove helped mask the taste of spoiled meat. More recently historians have pointed out that fresh game covered North America, but far-eastern spices did not. Use of spice, likely more a mark of celebration than privation, added to the exceptional nature of this post-midnight-mass tradition.

Irish French Meat Pie
Crust

- 2 cups all purpose white flour (plus a little)
- 2/3 cups plus 2 tablespoons Crisco shortening
- (I've used lard as they might have before my time – it's great)
- 1 1/2 tsp salt
- 4 tablespoons water or milk

Mix salt through flour. Cut shortening in until the mixture is mealy. You may use a pastry cutter, but two butter knives work well and it's how Genevieve did it. Add water or milk, one tablespoon at a time and work dough just until it becomes moldable. Do not over-knead.

Roll out half the dough between two sheets of wax paper or parchment paper. I lightly dust the paper with flour before I start. Place in bottom of a pie plate and roll out the other half for the top of the pie. Set aside to make filling.

Filling

- 2 tablespoons of butter
- ½ pound ground beef
- ½ pound ground pork
- One large onion
- 2 teaspoons ground cloves
- 1 teaspoon salt
- 1/2 teaspoon black pepper
- 1 1/2 cup mashed potatoes
- Potatoes, peeled, cut and boiled
- Milk
- Butter
- Salt
- Pepper

Mix up a mashed potato recipe of your liking. I like them lumpy. My mom made them very creamy. It's all on you – but make sure you use mashed potatoes, not just boiled potatoes as is common in other recipes. You'll thank me!

Slice onion and sauté in melted butter. Place in mixing bowl. Brown ground meat together, add to mixing bowl. Add spices and mix thoroughly. Add mashed potatoes and mix again. If you're concerned that it's not right, taste the filling. If you can't taste the spices, add a little more. The flavor will become more pungent after baking, but you don't want to start with a bland mixture.

Fill the pie shell with the meat/mashed potato mixture. Place the top crust over the plate and tamp down on the sides. I fold the sides up and over toward the center to get a little extra crust with each slice. Cut vents into the top and bake at 350 degrees for one hour. Serve with a green vegetable.

Vegetarian Irish French Meat Pie

If you managed to use fresh game and home-grown potatoes for your meat pie as the Franco-Americans would have done in the late 19th century, you could feed your family for pennies or less. My family recipe above ain't poor food, no matter how you slice it. To make matters worse for the vegan and vegetarian members of my family, the recipe calls for a fair quantity of dead animal.

Consequently, I modified the recipe. Here's how to make it for the non-violent imbibers in your home. For the vegan equivalent, substitute vegetable oil spread and oat milk for the dairy in this recipe.

Everything for this pie is the exact same as the above pie. BUT instead of using a pound of ground meat – use two pounds of mushrooms. I like to mix varieties. Remember to saute' mushrooms until most of the moisture is gone. The mashed potatoes hold the pie together beautifully. Sliced, this is one of the most beautiful pies on the table.

One last note about sauces – don't forget the gravy! There is never, ever, enough gravy. And good gravy can overcome the most humble dish. As G would say, "I never managed to get the gravy to outlast the chicken." She'd make gravy bites – gravy on cut-up pieces of toast. And loved popcorn gravy. Just like it sounds. Gravy poured over popcorn.

My soon-to-be child-in-law, Amy, makes vegan gravy with vegetable bouillon and oat milk. I kid you not – delish! Make a roux with flour and olive oil. Add equal parts bouillon and oat milk and let it simmer to thicken. Amy uses this gravy to make vegetable pies. They come together just like a chicken pie and – literally – are just as delicious. You can use any and all vegetables in this faux chicken pie. I like to use onions, celery, carrots, spinach and peas. It's chef's kiss worthy!

Chapter Eighteen

Maine Home Cooking

The only wicked-impoverished people I met – who ate food I'd like to eat – grew up growing their own food. Farmers, gardeners, urban planters and other types of agrarians supplemented their diets with food they cultivated on their own.

The recipes they supplied are well worth trying. Mixed in among those recipes are foods that some poor kids grew up eating but were glad to leave behind. Still, fresh broccoli from a garden or chickens from the chicken farm could go a long way to making a hearty meal that tasted darn good, too.

Here's just a little smattering of goodness that folks from Maine wanted to share.

If parents worked day jobs and came home to cook, canned soups or other prepared foods could be a time and energy saver.

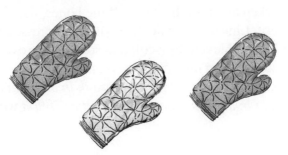

Let's start with a recipe from Betsy Garrold, lobbyist for farmers and tireless advocate for universal healthcare.

Maine Maple Syrup Baked Beans

- 2 lbs. yellow-eye or soldier beans
- 2 onions
- 2 tsp salt
- ½ lb. salt pork (optional or thick bacon as a substitute)
- 2 cups Maine maple syrup
- Enough water to cover beans

Rinse beans then place in a crock pot and soak overnight. Water should be a half inch over the beans. The next morning, bring the pot to a boil, but only until the skins peel back. Add onions, pork, and maple syrup; stir well and cook in a crock pot on high for several hours. Add salt and stir again, cook the rest of the afternoon.

Chicken & Broccoli Bake – Siblings Horrified

Julie from Skowhegan sent me this recipe for a dish her mom would make for a special treat. She told me that her sisters were horrified that she shared the recipe – I get it. I can't believe how much Rice-a-Roni I ate as a kid. (Thankfully, my mom stopped making boxed foods after the 1980s).

Julie explained the recipe this way: "We generally ate VERY bland foods, and this was quite creative and flavorful relative to the usual!"

- 2 lbs chicken legs and wings
- 2 cups cooked rice
- Broccoli, fresh for frozen
- Can cream of mushroom soup
- Mayonnaise (½ cup or so)

Boil the chicken and pull the meat off the bones. (Save bones and water for stock). Line a casserole dish with rice, pressed flat like a crust. Layer in the chicken, broccoli and soup, twice over, and bake. *"When mom was feeling particularly creative she would add mayo to the cream soup."* Bake at 350 for no more than 30 minutes. *"When I was struggling in my 20s I made it a few times but it was never as good as hers!"*

Shanna's Spiced Lamb Cabbage Rolls

Not every dish in Maine comes from Native-American or Franco-American roots. Maine's rugged coast and deep seaports drew mariners and their families from all over the world. At one time in the 19ᵗʰ century, the port downeast of Wiscasset had nearly a dozen languages represented in the schools. Shanna's dish, popular with eastern Europeans, may or may not have been common in her hometown of Lubec. But if Shanna's making it, it's a Maine dish now.

- 1 large head green cabbage – use the ten largest outer leaves whole, as directed below
- 1 lb. ground lamb
- 1 cup cooked brown rice
- 1 ½ inch ginger root, peeled and diced
- 4 large cloves of garlic, minced (save a little of this for the broth)
- 1 large, sweet onion ,finely diced (reserve half for broth)
- 1 egg
- 1 peeled, diced carrot
- 3 cups chicken broth (Shanna prefers Better Than Bouillon brand chicken stock – PS so do I)
- 1 tsp cinnamon (plus a sprinkle for broth)
- 2 tsp ground cumin (plus a sprinkle for broth)
- 2 tbsp parsley (plus a sprinkle for broth)

Steam entire cabbage head to soften outer leaves, until pliable enough to remove leaves without tearing. Remove 10 outermost leaves, cut out thick stem part and set aside (you can shave this down so that there is still a thin membrane left to keep the leaf whole). In a large bowl, mix lamb, spices, onion, garlic, ginger, egg, and cooked brown rice. Divide mixture into six oblong balls. Place in individual cabbage leaves and roll. Pour chicken broth into a dutch oven, casserole dish or covered skillet. Place cabbage rolls in the broth. Sprinkle the top with reserved onion, carrot, shredded leftover cabbage, parsley, cinnamon and cumin. Cover the pot. Bake in 350-degree Fahrenheit oven for one hour – or simmer on stovetop for a half hour. Serve warm in a bowl with broth.

According to the State of Maine, Maine produces 99 percent of the blueberries in the United States. When my kids were babies, Mrs. Lamb lived next door. Older than dirt, her family had been in Maine for generations and she shared the family blueberry cake recipe. Never use frozen berries for this. Oh, and you're welcome.

Mrs. Lamb's Blueberry Cake

- 1cup washed and dried blueberries – fresh, not frozen!
- Zest of ½ lemon
- 2 eggs
- 1 cup sugar plus a tablespoon
- 1 stick of butter
- 1 teaspoon vanilla
- 2 cups flour
- 2 teaspoons of baking powder
- ½ teaspoon salt
- ½ cup milk

Cream butter and sugar together. Beat in eggs. Add vanilla. In a separate bowl mix all the dry ingredients. Add the dry mixture to the sugar, butter, eggs and vanilla and mix well. Should be thick. Add milk until it becomes a cake batter consistency (you might need a few splashes more of milk). Add lemon zest and stir. Then gently fold in blueberries. Careful not to crush any.

Put into a greased cake pan and sprinkle the top with the last tablespoon of sugar. Bake at 350 degrees for 30 minutes or more – depending on the size and dimensions of your pan. Cake is done when a toothpick inserted into the center comes out clean.

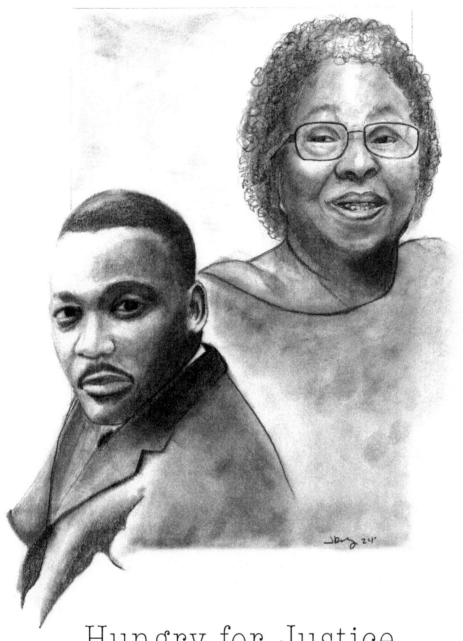

Hungry for Justice

Chapter Nineteen

Dinner Fit for a King

"When women escaped slavery, they had only two things, quilt patterns and recipes."

~ Cynthia Sawyer

A shy teen, Cindy Sawyer hid in the bedroom when Martin Luther King, Sr. (Daddy King, as they called him) and his grandson, Martin Luther King III visited her home.

It wasn't the first time that members of the nation's most iconic civil rights family visited the Sawyers' Richmond, Indiana home. Before his assassination, MLK, Jr. would drop by to confer with George Sawyer, an eastern Indiana attorney, civil rights leader and founder of African American studies at Earlham College. Still, it wasn't until after MLK, Jr.'s mother, Alberta Williams King's assassination, that King's extended family journeyed to Indiana and dined at the Sawyer home. There they enjoyed the loving embrace food and fellowship provide.

Earlham College, founded in the mid-nineteenth century by religious leaders who wanted to educate their children in their Quaker culture, eventually opened its classrooms to the public. Earlham expanded their mission of spreading enlightened thought, regardless of the students' religious affiliation. Earlham became the second-largest Quaker college in the world and the first and largest co-ed Quaker school of higher education.

Earlham's inclusive nature made it the perfect environment for progressive thought – and for progressive thinkers like George Sawyer. So much so, a century-old scholarship fund was renamed for Geoffrey Sawyer, George and Jackie's 12-year-old son who passed away from a life-long condition.

Family pictures pepper the shelves and tabletops of the Sawyer home. Framed photos of the children are interspersed with pictures of MLK, Jr. and Professor Sawyer leading public discussions for mostly white audiences. As a child, Cynthia remembers a picture of MLK, Jr. hung on the wall. "It was one of those pictures with eyes that seemed to follow you wherever you went in the room. I grew up thinking MLK, Jr. watched over us."

While Earlham embraced freedom and openness, much of Richmond proper did not. The Sawyer family often felt imperiled. So much so that during at one racially charged time and in reaction to bomb threats made against the community in general and the Sawyer family in particular, Jackie took the children and left home for a week.

On the night that a gunman shot and killed MLK, Jr. while standing on the balcony of the Lorraine Motel in Memphis, Tennessee, George Sawyer prepared to leave the house and attend an action with other outraged and grieving leaders. Jackie pleaded with him not to go. George, unwavering, was headed for the door when the phone rang.

Cynthia recalled, "It was grandma telling him, 'Do not leave that house.'" Cynthia's face wearing the same relief her mother's may have had that night, added, "He stayed home."

The United States spent years mired in turmoil. Bobby Kennedy, the students at Kent State, thousands of arrests and protests, the climax of the Vietnam War, and more mark a decade filled with chaos. Jackie saw all that fear and cruelty as part of a bigger plan to destabilize American communities despite continuing calls for equality. "The horror was disruptive."

In 1971 and '72, George and Jackie took their children to live in Kenya. The woman who had been delivered by midwives at her grandmother's house in Richmond, Indiana went with her husband and a group of American teachers to run African schools established by the Quakers. Earlham College Libraries have a link to a manuscript series about the program. It's in the endnotes with the other citations for *Humble Pie*.

While at the Harambee Schools, Jackie remembers that people were eager to speak with them. Sometimes people would stare at them, remarking, "These are the descendants of slaves that were taken to America." Jackie, a woman intimately connected to civil rights martyrs, paused and let the gravity of that statement settle. Then she added, "We felt very welcome. They wanted to know what we were doing there. The students were very interested in what was going on, what we did, what we ate."

I understood. I asked what they ate while they were in Kenya.

Jackie answered, "Well, at the market we didn't see what we get here. But they had these little biscuit things. They were very doughy. They were great."

I did a web search for "doughy Kenya biscuit things" and found several sites. All have lovely recipes. Some flavored with cardamom or cinnamon. It appears they're called "Baa." I don't have any original recipes to share, but I left some links in the bibliography.

Upon their return, George settled back into his African American Studies programs at Earlham and continued his civil rights work – incorporating the efforts of Daddy King as he struggled to continue his son's legacy. Shortly after Alberta's assassination, George told Jackie that Daddy King and his grandson would be coming for dinner. Her first thought, after those years of calm acceptance in Kenya, was, "Oh my gosh, he gets in a lot of trouble."

I asked if she was afraid to have Daddy King. She replied, "I was a little concerned." In those days, Jackie's job – protecting the children – occupied her mind all the time. "I'd think to myself, *Dear Lord, let me take care of the children so they won't be attacked*. People watched our house from across the street. They would just stand there and stare at it."

Jackie resists the temptation to conflate today's reactions to racial tensions and white supremacist crimes with what was happening in the early 70s. "In this day, people don't have passionate causes for which anger is not attached." She laments the loss of "A non-violent resistance: passion and purpose and a cause without volume attached." She looked at me earnestly and asked, "Why aren't there teach-ins anymore?"

When Daddy King and his grandson arrived, they had several bodyguards in tow. She vividly recalls preparing dinner with four large men overseeing her in the kitchen, "taking a teaspoon of everything and tasting it." The Sawyers' entire community contributed to the meal. Because so many had prepared different dishes in their own homes, Daddy King's security detail considered the possibility that every dish might be suspect. Each of those four men felt so committed to protecting MLK, Jr.'s family – especially after his mom's assassination – that if someone attempted to poison them the guards would have died instead.

The meal prepared to comfort the King family patriarch and his grandson consisted of sweet potatoes, corn bread, macaroni and cheese, pumpkin pie, sweet potato pie and collard greens. Proudly, Jackie proclaimed those weren't just any greens. They were prepared by her sister-in-law, Edna. "Edna was the queen of greens!"

Edna's recipe had been handed down to Donald, the oldest living Sawyer brother. He has passed that recipe on to us.

That evening's macaroni and cheese came from a neighbor and the recipe did not survive. We'll have to settle for my recipe and one more profound observation from Jackie. "It's all different when it's done for a cause. Their coming to visit; it was a cause. And the cause was defiance. Our whole community made the meal. Right down to the 'Defiance Macaroni and Cheese!'"

In honor of Jackie and her remarkable courage hosting the remnants of a martyred family, I will forever call our family favorite, "Defiance Macaroni and Cheese."

Jackie remembers Martin III as a painfully quiet but extremely polite boy. He'd just lost his grandmother, but he still remembered to say, "thank you." The only part of the meal Jackie made that night was the corn bread. Cynthia says she's always made the best corn bread. It starts out like so many others – with Jiffy boxed corn bread mix. But Jackie adds a flair. "It needs sweetener."

- 2 boxes Jiffy instant corn bread mix
- 2 eggs
- 2/3 cup milk
- 2 tablespoons white sugar (unless you've got some brown sugar in the house)

Bake at 400 degrees until inserted toothpick comes out clean.

Greens

As handed down to Don by Edna the Greens Queen. Don says that it goes with everything and anything – or can be eaten as a whole meal. He pairs it with turkey, steak, ribs, chicken, burgers and meatless alternatives, too. Don wants to remind you that because this recipe has no "real" measurements you must let your spirit guide you. The meat amounts are a guestimate, and you can use all of one kind or the other, if necessary.

- Mixture of collard (mostly), mustard and turnip greens
- 2 to 3 ounces of jowl bacon
- 2 to 3 ounces of cottage butt (pork shoulder)
- Lowrys seasoned salt
- Cracked black pepper

Cook everything (except spices) all together on a stove top. After about a half hour add the seasoned salt and the pepper to taste.

Here are a few recipes for the delicious food Cynthia made for me earlier this year when my friend, Max Goller, and I visited the family in Richmond. Cynthia, her youngest brother Michael, Jackie and I feasted on fruit, chocolates, a charcuterie board, sandwiches, cookies and the most wonderful lemonade I've ever had.

Chicken Salad

3 cups cooked and shredded chicken (or a whole rotisserie chicken (BJs and Costco are best – cut or shredded into small pieces)

- 1/2 cup celery, diced small
- 1 medium shallot, diced small
- 1/2 cup (or more) mayonnaise
- 1 ½ teaspoon Dijon mustard
- 1 teaspoon dried dill
- 1 teaspoon garlic powder
- 1/2 teaspoon salt or Goya's Adobo
- 1/4 teaspoon black pepper

Instructions:

This recipe is best made when tasting happens with each addition of an ingredient, especially since the meat from rotisserie chickens varies in amount and you may not get all three cups. Some people enjoy it more oniony than garlicky, so make it to your taste. Add more mayo if the salad looks too dry.

In a large bowl, combine the chicken, celery, shallot, mayonnaise, Dijon mustard, dill, salt/ Adobo, and pepper. Stir until well combined. Serve immediately or refrigerate for later.

Serving suggestions: sandwiches with provolone cheese, lettuce, and tomato or simply scoop onto salad greens.

Homemade Lemonade As a special gift –
a specialty of the Sawyer house!

- The juice of 6 large lemons (freshly squeezed is a must)
- 10 cups of water, divided
- 2 cups of granulated sugar

Instructions

Simple syrup: Put 2 cups of granulated sugar and 2 cups of water into a saucepan. Stir sugar and water for a few seconds until sugar begins to dissolve. Place saucepan over medium heat. When it begins to bubble on the edges, syrup should be clear and not cloudy. Instantly remove from the heat. (Be sure to remove from heat before syrup begins to turn brown).

Lemonade

Put 8 cups of water into a pitcher. Add freshly squeezed lemon juice. Add ½ c. simple syrup. Keep some spare lemons nearby. Stir and add additional juice, sugar and water to taste.

Leftover simple sugar stores in an air-tight container for 3-4 weeks.

Serve over ice cubes.

Jackie's Fried Chicken

- 3 lb. whole fryer broken down into 8 pieces
- ½ cup all-purpose flour (some remaining seasoned flour will be used to make a pan gravy)
- 1 tablespoon Lawry's Seasoned Salt
- Salt (optional)
- Pepper
- One inch of vegetable oil in a lidded saucepan

Wash chicken pieces well in cool water. Roll pieces of chicken into all-purpose flour. Lay out chicken on wax or parchment paper. Lightly shake salt (optional) and pepper on floured chicken pieces. Generously season floured chicken pieces with Lawry's. Lawry's is a must.

In a lidded sauté pan, pour one inch of vegetable oil. Turn on stove to medium heat. When the oil begins to shimmer, it is ready for chicken. Carefully place all pieces into the shimmering oil. When a piece is golden brown on the cooking side, turn the chicken piece with tongs. When each piece is turned, cover the chicken with a lid. Cook for 20 minutes. After 20 minutes, check wings (they will cook first), when they are golden brown on both sides, pull them out and place them on paper toweling to drain. Do the same with the rest of the pieces, returning lid each time. The breast and thigh will be the last pieces finished. The complete cooking time is about 30 minutes.

Pan gravy

Season the remaining flour and slowly add that mixture to the hot pan drippings on medium heat. Constantly whisk while adding flour until smooth gravy is formed. If gravy is too thick, add water to thin.

We had Cynthia's chocolate chip cookies at our interview. They are so fantastic. We are grateful that she shared the recipe here. And her pumpkin pie? Well, it has been proclaimed over and over again, by strangers and family members alike, as the best pumpkin pie recipe ever made!

Big Chocolate Chip Cookies

- 1 c. (2 sticks) butter (must be butter, not substitute)
- ¾ c. white sugar
- ¾ c. light brown sugar
- 1 tsp vanilla or almond extract or both
- 2 eggs
- 2 ¼ c. all-purpose flour
- 1 tsp. salt (scant)
- 1 c. broken walnuts
- 1 ½ c. semi-sweet chocolate chips (brand name are best)

Instructions

Preheat oven to 350 degrees. Place softened butter into large bowl. Add white sugar, brown sugar and vanilla. Stir with a wooden spoon (do not use a hand mixer). Add vanilla and eggs. Stir well. Add flour, salt, nuts and chips. Stir. Place ½ c. cookie balls on 2 parchment paper-lined cookie sheets (I use an ice cream scoop.) Set 12 cookies on each sheet, placed with space between them. Cookies should be of the same size. Bake cookies for 20 minutes. Turn cookie sheets in the oven, halfway through baking, to ensure even baking. Cookies should bake only until set. They should still be soft and pale yellow/brown when removed. Cookies should be removed to a wire rack to cool. Be sure not to overbake these cookies. If overbaked they will be crunchy rather than soft and chewy. Makes 24 large cookies.

Cindy's Easy Pumpkin Pie

- 1 unbaked pie shell
- 15 oz pumpkin puree
- 14 oz sweetened condensed milk
- 2 large eggs
- ¾ teaspoon cinnamon
- ½ teaspoon salt
- ½ teaspoon ginger
- ½ teaspoon nutmeg
- ¼ teaspoon ground cloves (optional)

Instructions

Preheat oven to 350 degrees.

Combine pumpkin, milk, eggs. Stir. Add cinnamon, salt, ginger, nutmeg. Stir well.

Pour filling into pie shell. Bake for 30-45 minutes until knife inserted in center comes out clean.

Cover pie crust edge with foil if it is browning too quickly.

Chapter 20

Strangers in a Strange Land

Events around the world displace people. Wars, famines, acts of terror, dictators who abhor opposition, and cataclysmic climate occurrences all force people from their homes. According to the UNHCR, a United Nations Refugee agency, 110 million people fled their homes in 2023 – more than any other year on record.

A plurality of the global refugee count now resides in Europe with Turkey hosting more displaced persons than any other country on the globe. While the rest of the world assists millions, the United States lags. In 2022, the year Russia invaded Ukraine, UN figures put the number of refugees the U.S. granted asylum to at 25,465, while poorer countries collaborated to shoulder the needs of millions more.

Historically, the U.S. has greeted immigrants – to greater or lesser degrees – who have fled war-torn lands. Clearly, not all applied for asylum. Some walked across borders. Some came as visitors and stayed. Others came on work visas and transitioned into green card holders and naturalized citizens. My mother-in-law, Ana, worked on a navy base in the Philippines where she met a young sailor. They married and she shipped stateside with him when the U.S. Navy relocated him to California. Eventually her husband's tour of duty ended, and the couple moved to the east coast where they became chicken farmers.

Ana used to laugh about how peaceful farms looked at a distance, "Because it took so much work to keep them that way."

I asked her about her life during World War II. She told me that – looking back – she'd learned a great deal from her bouts with starvation during the Japanese occupation. "I learned to feed a family of six with just one pork chop" and the produce she grew in her gardens. I'm going to share Ana's Pancit recipe here – which she'd modified to accommodate her meager income as a farmer in Maine.

In the 1960s, Ana lived more than 300 miles from the closest Asian grocery store and traditional vermicelli rice noodles were difficult to find. She'd make her Pancit using packaged, instant ramen noodles – which were invented in 1958 – the same year her first child, Alan, was born.

I need to share a story Ana told me about war and hunger. Anacorita Borlasa grew up in a small village at the base of the Philippines' Mayon volcano. Japanese soldiers had vanquished the islands and – as is always the case in war – food was scarce. Ana remembered, "especially rice." As in most Asian nations, rice had been a major staple of their diet. Without it, people starved. Historians estimate that half a million people, or more, died of starvation or disease during WWII in the Philippines alone.

A primary-school-aged child, my mother-in-law got thin and frail. A Japanese soldier, probably not ten years older than she, would share his rations with her. They became friends. I asked her if, looking back, his kindness shocked her. "Of course not. He didn't choose the war any more than I did." And with her sweet Filipino accent she added, "War is Stupid." Although to pronounce it the way she did, I should write, "Stoopeed."

Ana's Pancit

About a cup of every fresh vegetable you can find. More of cabbage and other leafy greens, less of bell peppers or asparagus and other pungently flavored ones. Make sure to have onions, lots of onions, if available.

- Several cloves of fresh garlic (chopped finely)
- Several thin slices of fresh ginger (slammed – yes slammed)
- Cooking oil
- Meat from one raw pork chop – or more if you can afford it – sliced into tiny strips. Raw chicken works well too.

- Soy sauce, salt and pepper to taste
- 2 or 3 packages of Ramen Instant Noodles (or more – depends on how many mouths you have to feed)

In advance of cooking, slice all the vegetables length wise. In the case of carrots or other vegetables, slice on the diagonal. Slice the meat in advance, too. This dish cooks very quickly, so prepping your raw foods is essential. In a very large fry pan (or wok) add the oil, minced garlic and slammed ginger. Ana would take the slices of ginger, lay a large knife side-ways on top of a piece on a cutting board and slam down on the knife's flat side with the heel of her fist. The thinly sliced ginger would then splay out into fibrous pieces. She would throw these into the oil. She never chopped her ginger because the flavor would be too hot – too strong, even in tiny pieces. After cooking, she removed the slammed ginger from the food or cautioned us not to eat it if it ended up on our plates. Once the aroma of ginger and garlic tickles your nose, add the sliced onions (not chopped).

At this point add ramen noodles to a separate pot of boiling water. They cook fast, so you're nearly done.

Add the fresh vegetables, saving the leafy ones for last. When the veggies cook down a bit push them to the sides of the pan – you may need to add a little more oil in the center – and cook your protein. This works really well with raw cashews if you want a vegetarian/vegan option. Often, Ana would add about 1/3 cup of soy sauce at this point, but that's really up to you.

Drain the cooked ramen and toss in with the prepared veggies and protein. Grab plates or bowls and start eating.

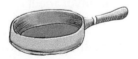

Perhaps it's easier for modern Americans to understand Ana's kind of immigrant – the young people who survived World War II and escaped beleaguered nations torn asunder as victims of the Axis/Allies fight. Ana, after all, hailed from an American territory, making her transition to the U.S. mainland easier to arrange. But not all World War II survivors who migrated to the U.S. came from allied territories.

Many, like a Virginia grandmother named Gisela, grew up listening to the sounds of American and British bombs falling on their home.

Her most vivid childhood memories were of her father shielding her and her sister from bombing raids that demolished her neighborhood.

Starvation during and after the second World War raged around the globe, with an estimated 25 million famine deaths in less than a decade. Gisela and her family escaped Eastern Germany long before the wall went up. So young at the time of their escape, her memories come back to her at strange times. Loud sounds in a movie theater will cause her tremble with fear. Often, the theatrical mimicking of explosions causes her to leave a film and go home.

Gisela and I spoke just after Russia invaded Ukraine. The cable news clips she watched on TV brought another Russian invasion back to her. "When we started our journey [to flee the Russian occupation of East Germany], we went on foot to Berlin to my dad's aunt. My father thought the capital would fall last. There are so many parallels to Ukraine. My mother painted her face black and made herself ugly to protect against rape. We hid in my aunt's basement."

Gisela remembers eating nettles in the woods to survive. When I interviewed her, she shared recipes for cooking with nettles that she'd found on the internet, but none that she could remember from her days in the woods. Then there were no recipes. They ate only to survive.

Consequently, Gisela promised herself that she'd never eat nettles again. Thankfully, decades later. Gisela doesn't have to forage in the woods, either.

Gisela is now living her senior years in comfort. Because she has more than she needs, she helps others. Working with me quietly and privately, she buys clothes and shoes for children experiencing homelessness – children she'll never meet – but who live a life she profoundly understands.

When I spoke to Gisela about sharing cooking hints from her privation, she preferred instead to share a recipe for a dish she loves to make now. One from before the war, when the ingredients were plentiful. She doesn't remember having this dish again until after they escaped the woods and got to safety. Gisela now enjoys this soup – far, in both space and time, from the violence and turmoil foisted on her by world leaders she never met.

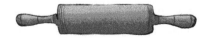

Gulaschsuppe
(Goulash Soup)

- 3-4 tablespoons oil
- 3 pounds of chuck roast, cut into 1/3 inch dice
- 3 medium onions finely chopped
- 1 tablespoon flour
- 2-3 tablespoons Hungarian sweet paprika
- 1-2 tablespoons tomato paste
- 1 tablespoon ground caraway seeds
- 1 teaspoon dried marjoram
- ½ teaspoon dried thyme
- 1 bay leaf
- 2 medium potatoes, peeled and cubed
- 6-8 cups of water
- 1 beef bouillon cube
- Salt and pepper to taste.

Heat oil in a sturdy pot and brown meat on all sides. Add onions and continue to sauté until onions are lightly browned. Add flour to thicken. Add water, bouillon cube and spices. Bring soup to a simmer. Cover and cook for about 1 to 1½ hours. Add potatoes and continue cooking uncovered for approximately 15 to 20 minutes, until potatoes are tender.

One night I went out to hear music. A singing duo, Momo and Emmanuel, shocked the small audience that had gathered to hear bands play from a makeshift stage. Neither performer knew each other when they fled the Democratic Republic of Congo (DRC), but danger at home and a search for security abroad led them to find each other and to share their talents.

Back in the DRC, Momo – a young woman in her twenties, lived a dual life. In the evenings she sang. She sang beautifully. Local embassies hired her to perform at various events. She brilliantly learned other languages and used her remarkable voice to portray soulful versions of national anthems that were not her own.

During the day, because of her desire to help the women in her own country, Momo worked to improve women's access to healthcare.

A law student, her activities drew the ire of political leadership and, eventually, the government targeted her. They arrested and tortured Momo. She became a political prisoner in her own land.

Following months of torment, employees at one of the embassies where she'd performed helped her to escape. She emigrated to the U.S. as an asylum seeker.

Momo can never go home. She faces constant reminders of what she's lost. Momo's mom died recently – having lived nearly a decade without seeing her daughter.

Emmanuel's dad, a minister, agreed to broker a peace deal during the civil conflicts that ravaged their homeland. He and other members of the clergy journeyed to meet with warlords. The peace delegation was ambushed and executed. Emmanuel's mom went to the authorities, certain that they were involved. Within weeks, she, too, was dead. Emmanuel lived in an orphanage with his siblings for six years, until he turned eighteen. As soon as he could leave on his own, the young musician fled to South Africa.

Emmanuel studied music his whole life. As a child, his father – a musician as well – told him that God and music would be his refuge. In South Africa he received rigorous formal training and expanded his talents. An accomplished performer and composer, Emmanuel's boundless talents created opportunities.

Offered a job at a music school back in Brazzaville, he tried to move home to be with his siblings. A wanted man, Emmanuel was arrested and threatened with life in prison, or worse. Again, Emmanuel escaped. When the authorities learned he'd slipped away and fled the country, they murdered the man who had helped him escape. Initially settling in Paris, Emmanuel had relatives in the United States. He hopped a plane and applied for asylum.

Emmanuel's passion for music introduced him to Momo – a fellow refugee – here in the United States. They adopted each other as siblings and started a musical journey together.

Life in the U.S. is difficult for asylum seekers. They don't qualify for public assistance and often must wait months to get a work visa. Without family or friends, many refugees have no way to feed or shelter themselves. Many states bar refugees from seeking help at food banks, even though the food is free.

Luckily for Momo and Emmanuel, Congolese enclaves exist in various parts of the country. There, kinsmen may be treated as family. Assistance from their fellow other migrants and from actual family members helped the duo survive. Fortunately for Momo and Emmanuel, they could share their vast musical talent with audiences who offered food and other support.

Food is more than sustenance. It is a form of communication, an expression of love. I asked Momo and Emmanuel to teach me to cook their favorite meals. Momo and I discussed the availability of food back in her home. She shared her dismay that food in the U.S. remained locked behind gates.

She also spoke of fufu. Fufu is a bread made from plantains (a fruit larger, but similar in appearance to a banana). The plantains are boiled, then ground into a flour-like meal. At an international market, I purchased a package of fufu mix to prepare for dinner one evening. I told Momo and Emmanuel that I wanted to try making food that tasted *like home*.

Momo gave me the recipe for Congo Stew. She and Emmanuel chuckled as they explained that they had invented the name for the dish. They said that they'd eaten a similar stew their whole lives, but it had no American name.

The original recipe calls for goat meat – a regular staple in both Momo's and Emmanuel's childhood homes. If I lived in a more urban setting, I'd have been able to get some.

Emmanuel stressed that the type of protein used was not the most important aspect of this particular concoction. "It must have two meats. Any two meats of your choosing. The stew cannot be made from just one type of animal."

I don't know if I made it right. Or if Momo and Emmanuel were just being kind when they said it tasted the way it should. That said, this recipe can be less expensive to make if you have time to stew the meats all day. Long cooking times allow for the use of less-tender and consequently less-expensive cuts. Root vegetables make up the rest of the dish. Extravagant additions like tomatoes can be used when the harvest season allows.

One last hint from Momo – whether you buy fufu mix or make it from scratch – be prepared to beat it for as long as five minutes to get the consistency correct. It's no surprise that fufu is much easier to make if you have an electric mixer nearby.

Congo Stew

- 1 pound of either beef, pork, goat, mutton (poultry not advised, but what the heck).
- 1 pound of a beef, pork, goat, mutton – but not the one you've already selected.
- ¼ cup of fat of some kind. Butter or bacon fat works beautifully, but any rendered fat will do.
- Root vegetables to include:
- Turnip
- White potato
- Sweet potato
- Yam
- Onion
- Squash of any kind to include:
- Pumpkin
- Butternut
- Acorn
- Additional vegetables you may have:
- Tomatoes
- Leafy greens to include:
- Spinach
- Kale
- Swiss Chard
- ¼ c flour
- 1 teaspoon salt
- 1 teaspoon pepper
- 3 bay leaves – if you have these ingredients available.

Chop the meat into small cubes. Combine flour with salt and pepper. In a bowl, coat the meat cubes with flour mixture.

In a large pot, melt the fat and add chopped onions. Caramelize the onions.

Add the dusted meats to the pot and brown. This can be done over a moderate heat. If cooking outside, be sure that you wait for all the coals to burn down without active flame, or you'll scorch the fat you're using.

Once the meats are browned, add water until the contents are entirely covered. Add tomatoes and bay leaves if you have them. Cover the pot and simmer for 2 hours. Add washed, cubed root vegetables and peeled squash and simmer another two hours. If you are adding leafy greens, do so at the 4-hour point and cook thirty minutes more. Remove the bay leaves and serve with fufu or over rice.

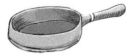

My buddy, Chef Archie – you'll meet him shortly – weighed in on the role of invasion, violence and various refugee movements on world-wide culinary diversity.

"It's hard to imagine a corner of the industrialized world that hadn't felt the influence of eastern cuisine. At one time, the sun didn't set on the British Empire. Consequently, everything from India Pale Ale to Tikka Masala has permeated the palates of the other regions that the Brits colonized over the centuries."

Chapter 21

Chop Suey or Goulash

Depending on the part of the country you hail from, you've likely grown-up eating either Chop Suey or Goulash. According to the website, *Fun Food Frolic* – American Chop Suey was named after a Chinese dish that came to the U.S. during the 1800s when thousands of Chinese immigrants emigrated to build the railroads.

The term sounds like a variation of tsap seui in the dialect spoken by these immigrants and translates loosely to mean, "various leftovers."

Now, totally Americanized, the dish is seldom made with leftovers. Instead, the meal has morphed into something like an Italian favorite, Spaghetti Bolognese. Outside New England, American Chop Suey is more commonly referred to as Goulash. The Passionate Foodie website claims that it is named after Hungarian Goulash, another dish whipped up from leftover ingredients.

While working on this book, I found that nearly everyone recalled eating a dish like this – by one name or the other – while growing up. I've included a few of those recipes here.

Karen Damborg of Readfield, Maine sent along her mom's recipe.

"Her name was Peggy Brann Damborg. Since my mother put Worcestershire sauce in everything, there was probably some of that as well. Plus, salt. We ate this so often that I have never – as an adult – made it!

Once, my mother was in the hospital and my father decided to make it. He got in his head that it would be greatly improved with cheap cooking sherry. My brother and I gagged.

I have since learned that the name is a New England thing. In other parts of the country, it is called Goulash and has green peppers added. I don't recall a green pepper ever entering our house."

American Chop Suey

- 2 cups cooked macaroni – or more depending on family size
- Half a pound to a whole pound of hamburger
- 1 onion, diced
- 1 can tomato sauce (she didn't specify size of can)
- 1 can tomato soup

Brown onion and hamburger. Stir in macaroni, tomato sauce and soup. Heat until hot.

Genevieve's American Chop Suey

We had Chop Suey with green peppers when I was a kid. I used to pick them out. We called it American Chop Suey. Just a reminder, my mother's recipes often called for some of something. The amount was subjective depending on the ingredient. Some salt was a pinch or so. Some sugar was about a half cup.

- 1 lb. ground beef
- 1 onion chopped
- 1 green pepper chopped
- "Some" oil
- One small can of tomato paste
- A 16 oz box of elbow macaroni
- Salt and pepper

Boil the noodles until cooked. Drain and set aside. Sauté onion in oil, brown ground beef. Add chopped peppers. Cook a little longer, then add the tomato paste. Use the can to measure a can full of water and stir into make a sauce. Mix in the cooked noodles.

Nan's Goulash

This recipe came with no amounts. Well, except the lard – if you consider a dollop a unit of measure. Because of the sour cream, this looks like a stroganoff variation. Yet, the family called it goulash.

- Ground beef
- Onion
- Garlic
- Canned tomatoes
- Dollop of lard
- Honey or sugar
- Dry macaroni
- Bay leaf
- Sour cream
- Water
- Ketchup

Brown beef with onion, garlic and a dollop of lard. Drain when no longer pink. Add tomatoes and liquid, plus honey or sugar and dry macaroni. Add bay leaf and use enough water to cover ingredients. Cook until most of the liquid is absorbed and macaroni are tender, about 10-12 minutes. Stir frequently while cooking. Remove bay leaf and discard. Stir in sour cream. Remove from heat and season with salt and pepper to taste before serving. Top with ketchup if desired.

Matthew's Grandmom's Goulash

Matthew Anderson – a man I met at work – shared his grandmom's recipe. It seemed more like a Shepherd's Pie, but he called it goulash.

"It was mainly at the end of the week. Come Friday or Saturday night money was tight so she would grab instant mashed potatoes, a can of green beans, a can of carrots, and as much ground meat as she could. Throw it all together and put it in the oven. Poof! Like magic, we had dinner for two nights."

"On good weeks she would put some shredded cheese on top."

- One can green beans
- One can carrots
- Ground beef (as much as you can get your hands on)
- Box of instant mashed potatoes, prepared according to instructions

Mix the vegetables with the ground beef and cook it all together. Cover cooked mixture with mashed potatoes.

Granny's Goulash

One particular Spokane, Washington Granny ended up raising her grandsons when their parents died. This particular goulash recipe became a family favorite. Granny made it in an electric frying pan, but any old frying pan with a lid will do.

- 1 lb. ground beef
- 1 onion, finely chopped
- 1 green bell pepper, finely chopped
- 1 lb. dry macaroni
- Salt
- Pepper
- 1 jar Pace brand salsa – medium hot
- 1 bag shredded Mexican cheese

Brown the ground beef and drain the fat. Stir chopped veggies into the frying pan with the meat and cook until tender. Salt and pepper to your liking. Add the dry macaroni and enough water to cover the mixture. Cover and cook until all the liquid is absorbed. Add the jar of salsa and the entire bag of grated cheese. Mix it all together and serve.

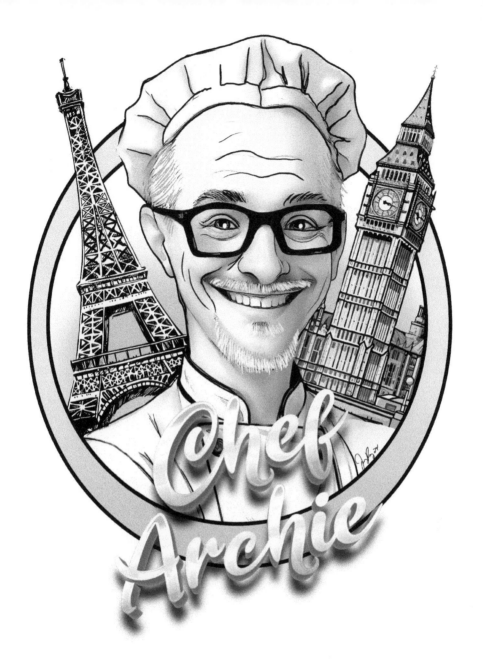

From Away

Tasty Affordable Treats

Crafted by Professionals

Chapter 22

When Pie is Your Love Language

Chef Archie Pie, aka *Archie the Pie Guy*, a classically trained food artisan and restaurateur, has cooked for the wealthiest patrons and the humblest diners. Trained first in France and later in the UK, he's prepared delicious meals in five-star restaurants and small village pubs. As a chef, he came to understand the intricacies of food chemistry, the value of fresh produce and proteins, the necessities of adequate storing and cooking temperatures as well as the expense of procuring it all.

Archie's recipes achieve the single common goal every cook strives to attain – excellent flavor. Secondarily, his concoctions look just as pretty as they taste. When Archie shifted away from working in other people's kitchens to owning his own restaurant, he was finally able to combine his love of cooking with his passion for the people who enjoy his creations.

At his own restaurant, Restaurant San Jacques, he would split his time between preparing meals and meeting the patrons who enjoyed them. Archie loved it. "Those were the greatest years of my life. People actually came to *my* restaurant and paid me to feed them – the greatest compliment any passionate chef/cook could be given." Many of those patrons became his friends. The chef's talents and charming personality caught the eye of producers at the BBC who included him in one of their most fanciful programs, *Mind Your Own Business*.

With Restaurant San Jacques, Archie had made his wildest dreams come true. Then a tragic accident stunted his career. The man who'd spent nearly every night of his adult life on his feet had to endure major surgery and lost mobility in his legs. He could no longer stand on the cooking line or run to the front of the house to greet his gourmet-loving guests.

After a lengthy recuperation, Archie found himself physically impaired but still overflowing with culinary ideas and passion. He needed a new outlet – one that showcased his flair for food and his penchant for people. Lucky for the Pie Guy, his housemate came to his rescue. "These days I adore cooking when my physical issues allow. My YouTube channel, the brainchild of my teenage daughter, Aimee, keeps me sane and active. Without her, I'd be doing nothing and awaiting expiration."

Archie and Aimee purchased tripods and some lighting equipment. They use his smart phone to film each episode. Prepping the recipes takes two to three hours but editing the video Aimee shoots takes the better part of two days. Days after the father and daughter team go into production, the finished video lands on his YouTube channel. There, people like me can watch and drool. On several occasions I've worked up the nerve to give his recipes a try. I've yet to be disappointed.

Like nearly every other living human being in the twenty-first century, I make friends with people over the internet. Sometimes they write to me first. Occasionally, I'm the one writing to them. A few years back, coincidental to planning this book – I started following this European chef on social media.

Pies are my love language. I make them to celebrate great things or simply to brighten dull days. I couldn't imagine anything more perfect than a man referring to himself as the Pie Guy. After implementing his instruction on a few of his creations, I decided to ask if he'd help with this book. I knew there'd be a lot of sad stories, and I wanted to provide a reward, at the end, to readers faithful enough to make it all the way to chapter 22!

I explained to Archie that all the proceeds would go to charity, and he jumped at the chance to help. When I learned more about his story, it all made perfect sense. His passion and patience – in the face of so much disappointment – are a perfect fit for our *Humble Pie*.

Nearly at the end, I've noticed – coincidentally – that pretty much every story in this book is about someone overcoming massive adversity to achieve a goal. In most cases it's a decent meal with enough calories to survive. Sometimes that comes with a bonus – enough flavor to evoke joy.

Archie generously has given us recipes that are super affordable (check out the onion recipes) along with a few his most popular – yet marginally more expensive – ones. Please, give them a try. All of the Pie Guy recipes have a QR code. When you scan it, your phone or tablet will bring you to his and Aimee's corresponding YouTube video.

The first is Chicken Pot Pie. It's one of the recipes that put Archie on the Pie Guy map! Unlike his onion soup recipe which costs less than £1 a serving, it's still a very reasonably priced and delectable meal with great presentation. Pot pies are how this pro-chef-turned-YouTube-sensation made his name. *(Remember – the Brits use weights rather than volumes. You can convert weight to volume using an online calculator).*

Special thanks to Aimee, who took off her video production cap and polished her transcription talents to transcribe all the recipes that Archie so generously shared with *Humble Pie.*

Chicken Pot Pie
By Chef Archie Pie

Yields 12 individual pies, 4.5" by 1.5"

- 2 lb. chopped, cooked chicken
- ½ cup each: onions, carrots, mixed bell pepper, celery
- 3 oz. butter
- 2 oz. flour
- 1 tsp. thyme
- 1 tbsp. each parsley and chives
- 2 minced garlic cloves
- 20 oz. chicken broth
- 7 ½ oz. heavy cream
- ½ cup mixed peas and green beans
- Salt and pepper
- 1 beaten egg to brush pastry tops

SCAN ME

Method:

Sauce:

Step 1: Melt the butter in a 3-4 quart pot.

Step 2: Add carrots, celery, garlic, peppers, onions, and herbs. On a medium flame, cook these vegetables until they are soft, stirring occasionally.   Step 3: Add the flour. Mix to a paste until all the flour has disappeared.

Step 4: Add the chicken stock in 3 parts, stirring to a paste and bring to a boil in between each addition.

Step 5: The sauce should now be thick. Add peas and beans.

Step 6: Bring to boil, now add heavy cream. Season with salt and pepper. Leave sauce for at least 4 hours in the fridge, or even better overnight.

Step 7: Mix chicken with sauce.

Pies:

Step 8: Roll out quarter inch thick bases for your pie dishes.

Step 9: Roll out tops. Try to use an object approximately the same size as your pie dish to cut out pastry tops.

Step 10: Fill each pie with chicken filling. Lightly brush rims with water.

Step 11: Put pastry tops on the pies. Seal rims with a fork or your fingers.

Step 12: Brush pies with beaten egg wash, and a shake of salt and pepper. Stab each pie twice, for ventilation.

Step 13: Bake for 30-35 minutes at 180C/350F. Limit pies to 4-6 per oven shelf.

Absolutely fabulous. Bon Appetit!

Cauliflower & Mushroom Bake
with Panko & Parmesan Crumb
By Chef Archie Pie

- 1 cauliflower (cut into small florets, boil for 6 minutes then drain and dry well)
- 5 oz. butter
- 2½ oz. flour
- 6 oz. sliced mushrooms
- 5 sticks celery chopped fine
- 1 large onion chopped fine
- 1 tsp. each parsley & thyme
- 2 garlic cloves minced
- 30 oz. hot milk or 50/50 milk & cream
- 8 oz. cooked bacon chopped
- 3-4 tablespoons each panko & parmesan
- salt & pepper to taste

Method:

Step 1: Melt 2 oz. of butter in a large pot.

Step 2: Add celery, onions, garlic, and herbs. Sweat until soft for 5 minutes.

Step 3: Add mushrooms and another ounce of butter.

Step 4: Add cooked bacon, stir fry for another 5 minutes.

Step 5: Turn off heat. Add flour. Mix to a paste until you can no longer see the flour.

Step 6: Turn on a medium flame. Add the milk in 4 batches, stirring and bringing to boil between each addition.

Step 7: Season with salt and pepper to taste. Reserve sauce for half an hour.

Step 8: Melt 2 oz. of butter in a frying pan.

Step 9: Over a low flame, add panko and parmesan until they have absorbed all the butter, then leave to cool.

Step 10: Place cauliflower in a suitable ovenproof dish and cover with sauce, then crumb. Bake for half an hour at 190C/375F. Flash for 20 - 30 seconds under the grill to brown.

Serve as a side dish, or as a main meal with buttered pasta.

Here are those onion dishes I promised you in Chapter 16 – The Omnipresent Onion.

Tomato Double Onion & Smoked Paprika Soup
By Chef Archie Pie

- 2 tablespoons olive oil
- 1 oz. butter
- 400g tomato pulp
- 3 tablespoons tomato puree
- 25 oz. beef or bvg or chicken stock
- 1 lb. sliced onions after peeling
- 1 teaspoon of smoked paprika
- Oregano & garlic powder – depending on your taste
- Dash brown sugar
- 1/2 teaspoon ancho chilies
- 2 bay leaves

Method:

Step 1: Fry half of the onions in half of the butter and oil until nice and brown for about 10 minutes. Stirring every two minutes. Sprinkle in brown sugar and finish caramelizing the onions.

Step 2: In a 4-quart pot, melt the remaining oil and butter, and cook the second half of the onions for 5 minutes, until they're just beginning to brown.

Step 3: Add all the spices. Stir fry on a low flame for 2-3 minutes. Step 4: Add some stock (4 tbsp) and continue cooking until it becomes syrupy.

Step 5: Turn the heat off and add flour to make a paste.

Step 6: Turn flame on low and cook for one minute, then add tomato paste.

Step 7: Add the beef stock gradually in four batches. In between each addition, stir in and bring to a boil.

Step 8: Add tomato pulp. Whisk this in and bring it to a boil. Simmer for 10-15 minutes.

Step 9: Add the caramelized onions, adding more brown sugar, check for salt and pepper and serve with croutons and a sprinkling of parmesan cheese.

Buttery Balsamic Baby Onions (Shallots)
By Chef Archie Pie

- 12-16 whole peeled shallots
- 2 oz. butter 1 bay leaf Sprig or 2 fresh rosemary 1 tablespoon sugar Few twists of salt and pepper
- 3 tablespoons balsamic vinegar
- 10" disc of parchment paper

Serves 4 (as a side dish)

Step 1: Peel the onions, but try to leave the root end slightly intact, so that the onions stay whole whilst cooking.

Step 2: In an 8" ovenproof frying pan, fry the herbs in the butter for 1 minute.

Step 3: Add the peeled baby shallots and let them cook for 2 minutes before sprinkling over with the sugar, adding a few twists of black pepper.

Step 4: Over a medium flame, cook the onions for 5 minutes, turning when necessary

Step 5: Once the onions start to take some color, add the balsamic vinegar, and cook for 2 minutes, turning all the time to ensure an even glaze.

Step 6: Cover with a lid of baking paper, and oven bake for 15-20 minutes on 180C/350F.

Step 7: Spoon over your finest grilled cheese sandwich for an amazing treat!

SCAN ME

In honor of our U.S. Thanksgiving Holiday, Archie made sure to include a recipe for turkey pie. Using leftovers, the cost per plated pie should be just less than a dollar a slice! As usual, check out his YouTube channel for step-by-step video instructions.

Fresh Turkey and Veggie Pies

- 2 lbs. cooked turkey
- 1 lb. frozen mixed vegetables, cooked
- 3 oz. butter or 3 oz. pork/bacon/beef fat
- 3 oz. flour
- 5 sticks celery
- 2 medium onions
- 40oz Turkey or Beef Stock (or 50/50)
- 2 cloves garlic
- 2 teaspoons dried parsley
- 1 teaspoon thyme
- 1 bay leaf
- 2 tablespoons tomato paste
- salt & pepper to taste

Archie didn't have time before we went to print to make a video for his famous Yorkshire pudding - although there are some wonderful recipes that have it as a feature. Still, it would be wrong not to include this tasty treat. Sorry to say, but, you're on your own!

.Archie's Yorkshire Pudding

- 4 oz. of beaten egg
- 4 oz. of milk
- 4 oz. sieved flour
- 1 tsp. veg. oil

Mix ingredients and rest in the fridge for one hour. Grease a shallow ½ inch hole tin (a muffin tin would work but only fill halfway. Popover pans are ideal). Place in a hot oven – 400 degrees – take out and pour in mixture. Back for 25 minutes. Makes 12 "pudds"!

Chapter 23

A Few Last Gifts from the Professionals

Chapter twenty-three – A Few Last Gifts from the Professionals

Jason Turner became a chef the old-fashioned way. He apprenticed. In elementary school, Jason knew he loved to cook. Fancy cooking schools and big city hobnobbing don't happen for kids like Jason. Instead, after he'd done a stint in the U.S. Marines, he went to work in central Pennsylvania kitchens, learning from small-town culinary experts.

Over the years, Jason changed kitchens and head chefs. He won awards and contests – distinguishing himself as one of the area's most accomplished chefs. Each successive move brought him closer to his dream of owning his own restaurant. It's a rare combination of things – a successful business owner and a full-time food artist. Jason realized that he preferred pairing flavors to managing financial assets.

Now, with his kids all grown, Jason lives and works on the west coast of Ecuador. Ten percent of the country lives on less than $4 U.S. a day. Jason grows the food that he cooks to feed his new community, and he loves it.

You might want to follow him on social media. (He's on my Facebook friends list.) If you like making a difference, he generally has a project or two that you can support.

For now, Jason's shared a few staples for your enjoyment. They are relatively inexpensive to prepare – especially so if you have a garden.

Basic Marinara

- ½ cup garlic
- 2 cups vegetable stock
- 4-6 cups roasted tomatoes
- 4-6 cups fresh tomatoes, chopped finely
- ½ cup tomato paste
- A handful of fresh basil, chopped finely (or 2 tablespoons dried)
- Olive oil (optional)

Cook garlic until translucent. (You may use oil, if needed). Deglaze your pot with vegetable stock. Add all the tomatoes, including paste. Bring to a boil, then reduce to a simmer. Let simmer 30 to 40 minutes, stirring to prevent sticking. Remove from heat, add basil, stirring to incorporate. Cool and can/freeze/refrigerate/use/store.

Veggie Stock

"This is a great way to use up vegetable scraps. You can make this while preparing vegetables or save the scraps in the freezer. Make the stock when you have enough scraps collected."

- 1 ½ cups onion scraps
- 1 ½ cups celery scraps
- 1 cup carrot scraps – no green parts
- 1/4 cup garlic scraps or 2 cloves
- ½ cup tomato scraps
- 6 cups water
- Oil

Place all scraps in a pot with small amount of oil. Sauté until they start to break down and darken. Add water. Bring to a boil. Reduce to a simmer and simmer 30 to 35 minutes. Strain. Cool. Can be used immediately or frozen.

Crisps and Cobblers
Filling

- 6 pints berries or fruit
- 1/3 cup sugar
- 2 tablespoons flour

Topping

- 2 cups sugar
- 2 cups flour
- 2 tablespoons baking powder
- 1 tablespoon salt
- 2 eggs
- Optional 1 tsp vanilla or other extract
- Melted butter

Combine dry ingredients, then add beaten eggs, mixing just until it resembles coarse cornmeal. Create fruit mixture and press into large, buttered dish or individual ramekins. Cover with thick layer of dough and drizzle with melted butter. Bake at 350 F until crusty.

From the Caribbean!

As a teenager, Bryan Landers and his family emigrated from the island nation of St. Lucia. Growing up around American cuisine, Bryan wanted to open a restaurant in the U.S. and share the flavors of his island home. B&L Caribbean Restaurant located in Carlisle, Pennsylvania has become one of the area's most popular eateries. Bryan and his specialty dishes have won people's choice awards, year after year, ever since his first bricks-and-mortar dining facility opened in 2021. Before that, Bryan had award-winning lunch wagons that were the hit of food festivals and community events.

Banana Salad
Made with green bananas

Not surprisingly, this dish features fruits and fish – everything you'd expect from a tropical island paradise.

- Hand of green bananas (that's what you might call a bunch)
- Assorted fresh vegetables
- Cod fish (or tuna)
- Mayonnaise
- Salt
- Pepper

Green bananas have a lot of starch, so you might want to add olive oil or vegetable oil to your own hands before you peel the hand of bananas. This way you won't get sticky while peeling. Place whole bananas in boiling water, add a teaspoon of salt. Boil about 25 minutes – don't let them get too soft.

While bananas are boiling, boil cod fish separately. (You may substitute fresh tuna). Cook vegetables. Use the veggies you like best. Cut bananas into one inch chunks. Mix bananas, fish and veggies all together and chill. Once the ingredients are cold, add black pepper and some mayo. If you like things a little spicy, you can add hot pepper.

The Irish Goodbye

I opened this book with tales from my family. Now, I'll close that way too. Some of the language in these last recipes my seem unfamiliar. I didn't modernize the references. I'm keeping it the way it was written. After all, if the woman who created this dish were still alive, she'd be more than 120 years old.

My mom's Aunt Martha died when I was in college. I loved her dearly. At the funeral, the priest said that he'd been called by the hospital at the point of her passing. He said that the doctor told him, "Martha Keady's heart failed." The priest then added, "I didn't believe him. I already knew that Martha Keady's heart never failed anyone."

Truer words, never spoke.

My Aunt Martha – my grandmother's sister – was a professional chef. Ironic, considering that she'd been one of the hungry Irish back in her youth. My Nana sent her money to join her in Boston. Martha only came to the U.S. to bring her sister home. Of course, that never happened. Mary refused, so Martha stayed.

Martha cooked in the homes of the wealthy. I remember my mom taking us to visit her at one of the Newport, Rhode Island mansions where she worked. The family was away and we sat in the formal dining room eating cheeseburgers and french fries. After lunch, we played in their elevator until my mom made us stop. I reached out to a cousin for some of my aunt's recipes. Jeanne shared this family favorite.

Chicken Veneziana

- 4 boneless & skinless chicken breasts dredged in seasoned flour
- Seasoned flour
- 1/3 cup flour
- ½ cup breadcrumbs
- Black pepper

- Granulated garlic
- 3-4 oz. prosciutto (Italian cured ham) sliced paper thin, trim fat
- 7-8 oz. fresh sliced mushrooms
- 1 tablespoon butter for sautéing mushrooms
- 1 cup (24-26) snow peas, clean & snip off ends
- ½ cup frozen peas, thawed
- 4 – 1/8-inch-thin slices provolone cheese
- Oil – just enough to sauté chicken
- 16 oz of cream and butter sauce (reduced/cooked while preparing chicken)

Heat sauté pan over medium heat with just enough oil to coat the bottom of the pan. Brown off chicken breasts in oil, approximately four minutes on each side. Season with pepper and granulated garlic. Set chicken aside and keep warm. Sauté prosciutto quickly on high heat, just enough to curl it. Sauté mushrooms on high heat. Use one tablespoon butter, season with pepper and garlic. Brown approximately 3-4 minutes. Prepare cream and butter sauce.

Cream and Butter Sauce

- ¼ cup sweet butter
- 2 ½ cups light cream
- 1 ½ cups heavy cream
- 1 egg yolk
- ¼ cup chopped fresh parsley,
- 1 ½ teaspoon granulated garlic
- ½ teaspoon black pepper

Melt butter until foaming. Be careful not to boil or let separate. Whisk in both heavy and light creams. Heat until lukewarm. Whisk in egg yolk, season with pepper and garlic. When chicken is ready – bring cream to a rapid boil. When thickening and mixture is reduced by approximately two ounces, add frozen peas.

Divide chicken, mushrooms, prosciutto onto four warm serving plates Top each breast with 1 slice of provolone cheese. Ladle each with four ounces of cream and butter sauce and arrange snow peas to the side. Brown under broiler for about one minute and serve.

Just Desserts

Welp, after five years, I finally finished *Humble Pie*. As I read and re-read it for editing purposes, I noticed something. I should have subtitled it, *Eyewitness Accounts of Survival*.

From page one, I cautioned that *Humble Pie* ain't no textbook. Although, I could have gone farther. Sure, it's got references in the back so you can see that I didn't make up my statistics. But, in addition to reporting on certain aspects of food insecurity in the U.S., *Humble Pie* is more like a memoir.

Please allow me to reverentially thank you for your company as I strolled down memory lane. I sincerely appreciate you reading about my experiences along the way.

Oh gosh, who else to thank…

There are so many.

Chad Bruce, my husband, who encourages me daily, also designed this book. Even after the editing process, this compendium of stories, first-hand accounts, recipes and references had to be formatted. I've written many books. Never has one been in greater need of direction, order and style. Like he does in so many other aspects of my life – he saw beauty in the mess and teased order and organization out of the rough.

Humble Pie wouldn't be a book if not for the stories of people I've met along the way. Some of them – Geralyn, Tom, Tonya, Max,

Melissa and Cristy – knew that their stories mattered because of the lived experience that flavored every aspect of their lives. Others – Jody, Betsy, Chris, Archie, Bryan, Jason, Jackie, Cynthia and so many others – turned their struggles into culinary triumphs. Meals to be celebrated and food as a celebration.

(If you've read this far, you know it contains dozens of first-hand accounts and recipes).

I'm also grateful to the folks who don't know that their stories are in here. People who struggled and with whom I've lost track.

Jeremy Ruby – your talent is superb. Your artwork softened the blow that a book about tragedy delivers. I'm humbled by the beauty you created to accompany my words as well as how masterfully you illustrated a humanity that encourages strangers toward empathy.

Lastly, to my editor, Cheryl Dunn Bychek. Goddammit – you're amazing. An editor is like the guy on the old Andy Williams show who had a table with tall sticks upon which he balanced plates. The plates stayed aloft if the man kept twisting the pegs to keep them spinning. Spinning the plates wasn't as impressive to me as knowing that he had to watch them all at once, to see which might fall next. Cheryl's ability to value my overarching message at the same time she finds a missing comma... well, she's second to none!

Bibliography

Who Actually Buys a Gold Toilet? Pasheva, Yana, 2021. https://slate.com/human-interest/2021/07/gold-toilet-corruption.html

Selina Wamucci, Ghana Spinach Prices, 2019. https://www.selinawamucii.com/insights/prices/ghana/spinach/

The World Counts, 2021. https://www.theworldcounts.com/challenges/people-and-poverty/hunger-and-obesity/how-many-people-die-from-hunger-each-year/story

Feeding America, 2021. https://www.feedingamerica.org/hunger-in-america/facts

Christopher Crosby, The Story of Maine Lobster, From Prison Food to Delicacy, Culture Trip, June 12, 2023. https://theculturetrip.com/north-america/usa/maine/articles/story-maine-lobster-prison-food-delicacy

Sandy Oliver, What you hear about lobsters and what's true, Island Institute, July 14, 2015. https://www.islandinstitute.org/working-waterfront/what-you-hear-about-lobsters-and-whats-true/

CIA World Fact Book, Infant Mortality rate, 2021. https://www.cia.gov/the-world-factbook/field/infant-mortality-rate/country-comparison

World Food Program USA, https://www.wfpusa.org/explore/wfps-work/who-wfp-serves/childhood-malnutrition/

USDA Food and Nutrition, Afterschool Programs. https://www.fns.usda.gov/cacfp/afterschool-programs

Urban Institute, Feeding America – Feeding Low-Income Children, October 2, 2010. https://www.feedingamerica.org/sites/default/files/research/latino-hunger-research/low-income-hispanic-children.pdf

3 Reasons the UAW is Having Success in Organizing Southern Workers, The Conversation, May 7, 2024. https://theconversation.com/3-reasons-the-uaw-is-having-success-in-organizing-southern-workers-with-two-mercedes-plants-in-alabama-the-next-face-off-228478

Irish Immigration to America, Claire Santry, 2024. https://www.irish-genealogy-toolkit.com/Irish-immigration-to-America.html

Safa Faruqui, Ten Rewards of Feeding Others, Muslim Hands, 02 July 2021. https://muslimhands.org.uk/latest/2021/07/benefits-of-feeding-the-poor-in-hadith-and-quran

Limestone Family of Three Dies in Fire, Sun-Journal, March 1, 2006. https://www.sunjournal.com/2006/03/01/limestone-family-3-dies-fire/

Space heater started fire that killed 7-yeah-old North Texas girl, authorities say, FOX 4 Dallas-Fort Worth, February 2024. https://www.youtube.com/watch?v=OCuQNhTAWBU

Family struck by tragedy again after home burns, Times Gazette, Irv Oslin, February 16, 2007. https://www.times-gazette.com/story/news/2007/02/16/family-struck-again-by-tragedy/19080133007/

The Conversation, Nearly half of all churches and other faith institutions help people get enough to eat, October 28, 2021. https://theconversation.com/nearly-half-of-all-churches-and-other-faith-institutions-help-people-get-enough-to-eat-170074

Soup Kitchens, Encyclopedia.com, https://www.encyclopedia.com/food/encyclopedias-almanacs-transcripts-and-maps/soup-kitchens

U.S. Cities Fact Sheet, Center for Sustainable Systems, University of Michigan, 2022. https://css.umich.edu/publications/factsheets/built-environment/us-cities-factsheet

Monique Allen, The Six Environmental and Health Benefits of Growing Your Own Food, August 2021. https://www.thegardencontinuum.com/blog/the-6-environmental-and-health-benefits-of-growing-your-own-food

Claude Belanger, French Canadian Emigration to the United States, Quebec History, Marianopolis College, August 23, 2000. http://faculty.marianopolis.edu/c.belanger/quebechistory/readings/leaving.htm

Sasha Chapman, Tourtiere, Britannica, July 18, 2018. https://www.britannica.com/topic/tourtiere

Brief History of SNAP, USDA Food and Nutrition Service, June 25, 2024. https://www.fns.usda.gov/snap/short-history-snap#:~:text=However%2C%20in%20fulfillment%20of%20a,of%20Food%20Stamp%20pilot%20programs.

As Food Stamps turn 60, four reasons to celebrate, Harvard Public Health, 2024. https://harvardpublichealth.org/policy-practice/food-stamps-are-turning-60-heres-why-we-should-celebrate/#:~:text=Signed%20into%20law%20on,a%20government%20program%20that%20works.

Clinton-Gore Accomplishments, The White House, 2001. https://clintonwhitehouse4.archives.gov/WH/Accomplishments/welfare.html

School Lunch Debt Statistics, Education Data Initiative, Melanie Hanson, January 9, 2024. https://educationdata.org/school-lunch-debt

Walter Parenteau, Tourtiere, The Canadian Encyclopedia, October 8, 2019.

https://www.thecanadianencyclopedia.ca/en/article/comfort-foods-from-canada

Culinary Lore, Food, Science, History and more, March 30, 2014. https://culinarylore.com/food-history:spices-used-to-cover-taste-bad-meat/

http://www.vegetablefacts.net/vegetable-history/history-of-onions/

LaMarche, Pat, Harrisburg is Stealing from Poor Kids to Fund Pregnancy Crisis Centers, The Bucks County Beacon, April 25, 2023. https://buckscountybeacon.com/2023/04/harrisburg-is-stealing-from-poor-kids-to-fund-crisis-pregnancy-centers/

State Fact Sheets: How States Spend Funds Under the TANF Block Grant,

Center on Budget and Policy Priorities, September 23, 2024. https://www.cbpp.org/research/income-security/state-fact-sheets-how-states-spend-funds-under-the-tanf-block-grant

14 GOP-led states have turned down federal money to feed low-income kids in the summer. Here's why, Jonathan Mattise, Geoff Mulvihill, Associated Press, February 16, 2024. https://apnews.com/article/states-rejecting-federal-funds-summer-ebt-8a1e88ad77465652f9de67fda3af8a2d

The Story of Food Not Bombs, Food Not Bombs, 2021. http://foodnotbombs.net/story_of_food_not_bombs.html

DRC: War in Ukraine Sparks Food Security Fears, Lauriane Noelle Vofo Kana, Africa News, August 13, 2024. https://www.africanews.com/2022/03/16/drc-war-in-ukraine-sparks-food-security-fears//

Urban Fruit for Urban Communities, Beattra Wilson, USDA, December 16, 2011. https://www.usda.gov/media/blog/2011/12/16/urban-fruit-urban-communities

USA for UNHCR, The UN Refugee Agency, 2024. https://www.unrefugees.org/refugee-facts/statistics/#:~:text=More%20than%20114%20million%20individuals,levels%20of%20displacement%20on%20record.

How Many Refugees are entering the United States? USA Facts, 2024. https://usafacts.org/articles/how-many-refugees-are-entering-the-us/

Demographics of Debt, Debt.org, Bill Fay, December 4, 2023. https://www.debt.org/faqs/americans-in-debt/demographics/

Hunting Season, Maine History Online, Maine Memory Network, 2010. https://www.mainememory.net/sitebuilder/site/182/slideshow/216/display?format=list#:~:text=Legislators%20continued%20to%20try%20to,hunting%20was%20banned%20until%201980.

Occupy Wall Street Begins, History, September 14, 2021. https://www.history.com/this-day-in-history/occupy-wall-street-begins-zuccotti-park

Amy McCarthy, Sour Dough is Having a Moment – Again, Eater, March 12, 2024. https://www.eater.com/24094642/sourdough-bread-trending-again

Onion History, National Onion Association, 2024. https://www.onions-usa.org/all-about-onions/history-of-onions/#:~:text=Many%20archaeologists%2C%20botanists%2C%20and%20food,or%20even%20writing%20was%20invented.

Research Starters: World Wide Deaths in World War II, The National World War II Museum, https://www.nationalww2museum.org/students-teachers/student-resources/research-starters/research-starters-worldwide-deaths-world-war

The Famines of World War II, Cormac O'Grada, Center for Economic Policy Research, 2023. https://cepr.org/voxeu/columns/famines-wwii

Chris Joe, Fried Chicken, CJ EATS recipes, July, 24, 2023. https://cjeatsrecipes.com/easy-fried-chicken/

The Geoffrey Sawyer Scholarship Fund, The New Association of Friends, 2014. http://www.newassociationoffriends.org/geoffrey-sawyer-scholarship-fund

Campus and History, Earlham College, 2024. https://earlham.edu/about/campus-and-history/

Aid starts flowing into Gaza Strip across temporary floating pier U.S. just finished building, CBS News/AP, May 17, 2024. https://www.cbsnews.com/news/gaza-pier-us-built-aid-flowing-israel-rafah/

RFE/RL, African Union Chairman says Putin's Grain Offer is not enough, Calls for Cease-Fire in Ukraine, June 28, 2023. https://www.rferl.org/a/african-union-chairman-ceasefire-grain-deal-insufficient-ukraine-putin/32524692.html

Quakers in Kenya: Friends Manuscript Series, Earlham College, September 21, 2023. https://library.earlham.edu/c.php?g=364359&p=5097449

Kenyan Style Biscuits, Mayuris Jikoni, May 11, 2012. https://mayuris-jikoni.com/2012/05/11/42-rolled-biscuits/

Kenyan Baa Biscuits, Mostly Food and Travel, Neha, October 18, 2023. https://mostlyfoodandtravel.com/kenyan-baa-biscuits/

Stealth Food Banks Serve the Undocumented, Food Bank News, July 14, 2020.

https://foodbanknews.org/stealth-food-banks-serve-the-undocumented/

Veg Chinese Chop Suey Recipe, Fun Food Frolic, Hina Guiral, December 13, 2022. https://shorturl.at/OkRpr

The Origins of American Goulash, The Passionate Foodie, January 6, 2023. https://passionatefoodie.blogspot.com/2023/01/the-origins-of-american-goulash.html

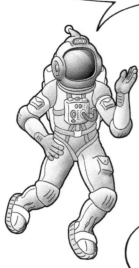

HI! WAM! THE SPACEMAN HERE...
Cosmic Ambassador of the Charles Bruce Foundation

WE PUBLISH ALL SORTS OF BOOKS AND USE THE PROCEEDS TO HELP ARTISTS OF EVERY STRIPE. SOME FOLKS GET GIGS THROUGH OUR AGENCY AND NEW OPPORTUNITIES TO EXPRESS THEIR TALENTS.

OTHERS HAVE MORE PRESSING NEEDS. WE ARE SMALL, SO WE JUST HELP THE BEST WE CAN.

I DON'T HAVE TO TELL YOU THAT IT'S LONELY IN OUTER SPACE. AS I PASS OVERHEAD, I SEE FOLKS IN NEED AND LOOK FOR WAYS TO HELP. IF YOU READ SOME OF OUR BOOKS - YOU'LL FIND WAYS TO HELP, TOO.

HERE ARE SOME OF THOSE TITLES WRITTEN BY PAT LAMARCHE THAT EXPLAIN THE INTRICACIES OF HOMELESSNESS. ALL PROCEEDS GO TO CHARITY BECAUSE ONLY A SUPERVILLAIN WOULD MAKE MONEY ON HOMELESSNESS.

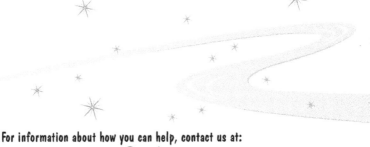

For information about how you can help, contact us at:
epicjourney10@gmail.com

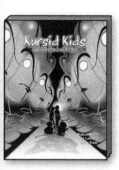

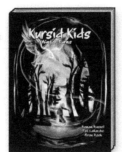

Kursid Kids
Winter Turns

Kursid Kids
For the Love of Pearl

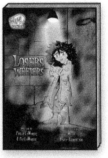

Losers
Weepers

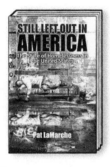

Still Left Out
in America

Priscilla and Her
Pals in the Park
(ages 5 – 9)

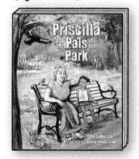

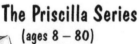

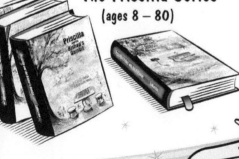

The Priscilla Series
(ages 8 – 80)

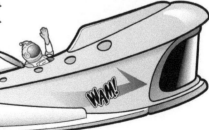

9 798988 181620